YOGA

a way of life

KU-485-485

YOGA
a way of life

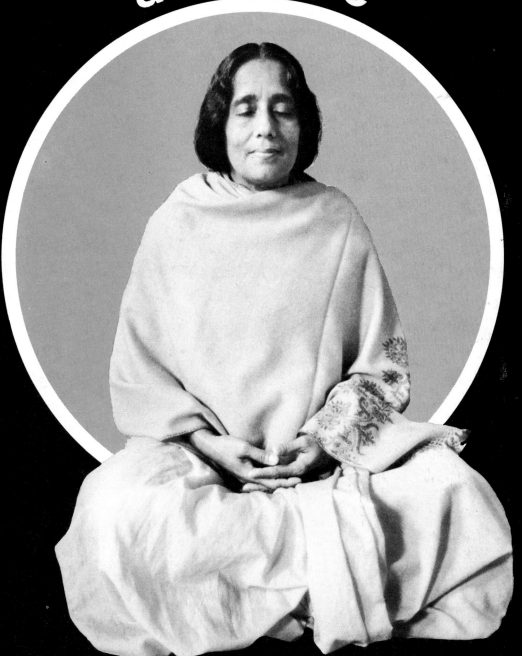

Ronald Hutchinson

Hamlyn
London · New York · Sydney · Toronto

Published by
The Hamlyn Publishing Group Limited
London · New York · Sydney · Toronto
Astronaut House, Feltham, Middlesex, England

© Copyright The Hamlyn Publishing Group Limited 1974
0 600 39268 6

Text set in England by London Filmsetters Limited
Reproduction in England by Colour Workshop Limited, Hertford
Printed in Spain by Printer Industria Grafica sa, Tuset 19,
Barcelona, San Vicente dels Horts 1974
Depósito Legal B-32207-1974
Mohn Gordon Limited, London

CONTENTS

INTRODUCTION

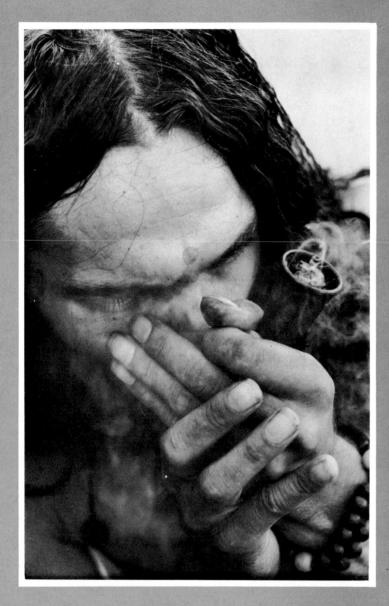

This is not Yoga.

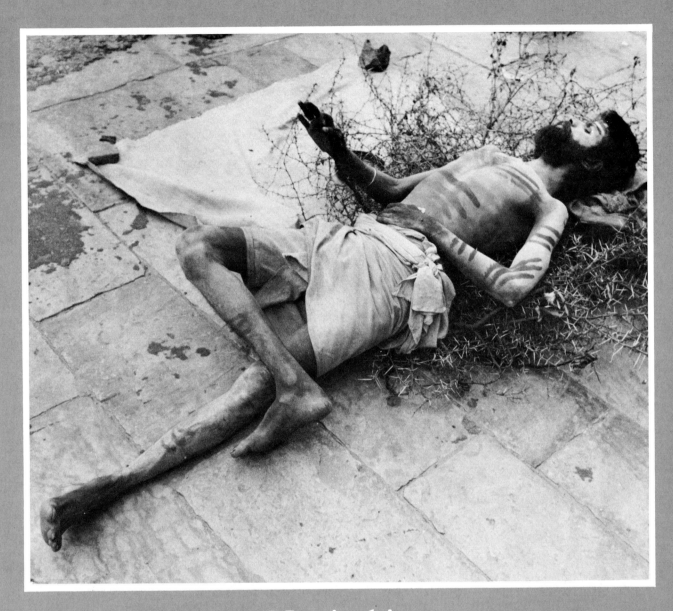

Nor is this.
So what the hell is it?
What is Yoga?

'Hear now
the wisdom of Yoga,
path of the Eternal and freedom
from bondage. No step is lost
on this path and no dangers are
found. And even a little
progress is freedom
from fear.'

Bhagavad Gita

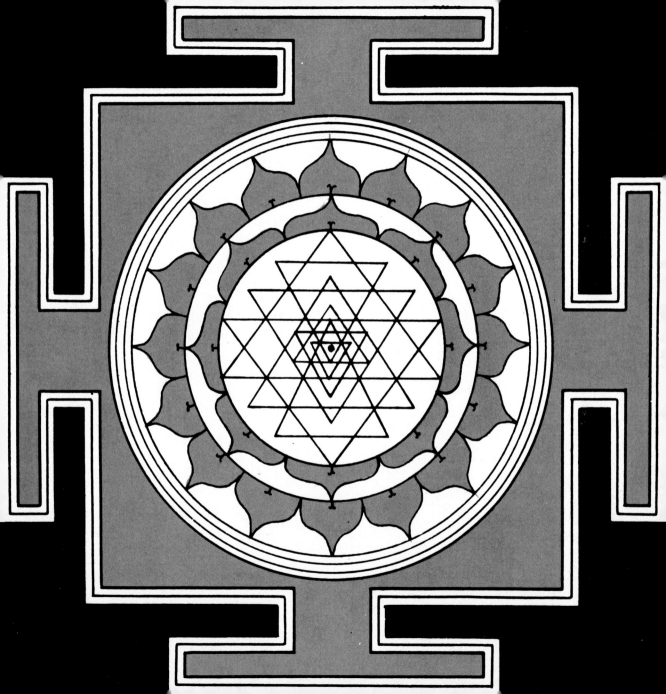

THE BEGINNINGS OF YOGA

In the valley of the River Indus, in what was then north-east India, a team of archaeologists under Sir Mortimer Wheeler discovered the remains of a civilization which, in its day, had been as powerful and as advanced as the Roman Empire or the Egypt of the Pharoahs. It even rivalled the fabled empire of the Incas of South America.

The 'Indus Valley dig' took place some fifty years ago but the finds were so rich that scholars are still working to evaluate their meaning. Amongst them were a number of seals depicting horn-capped figures sitting in positions which are too like advanced Yoga postures to be coincidence. This find suggests that Yoga existed long before the north of India was colonized by its Aryan invaders in 1500 BC, but until the Indus script has finally been deciphered one can only say that Yoga is so old that it dates almost into pre-history.

Yoga is without doubt the oldest form of personal development in existence and yet very little is known about its history. There are three basic reasons for this. The first is that the Indian mind has never been particularly concerned with the recording of history so that the distinction between actual event and religious legend has become blurred. The second is that knowledge, and Yoga knowledge in particular, was handed down by demonstration and word of mouth from teacher to pupil. Priests performed incredible feats of memory during rituals and even today there are those who can memorize the entire 2,400 stanzas of the *Ramayana*. With this tradition of memorizing it is not surprising that early written material is scarce. For thousands of years, then, Yoga was a secret technique, handed down only by direct tuition, and this tradition of secret teaching is the third reason for the lack of recorded history on Yoga. Being secret and keeping apart from the establishment priests and leaders of the times, Yoga developed the reputation of being "not quite nice to know".

At this point we should sort out any confusion between the yogi and the fakir. Lying on a bed of nails is essentially a fakir pursuit. Fakirs were originally wandering Muslim magicians who developed into a caste of street entertainers and beggars. They adopted some Yoga techniques but their aim was only commercial and they had none of the interest in finding a better way of living or of understanding the cosmos that has always been the

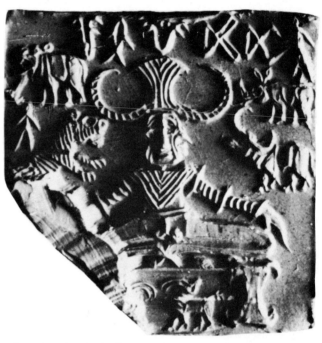

Seated yogi-style, the figure on this ancient Indus seal (*circa* 2500 BC) found at Mohenjo-daro dates Yoga almost into pre-history.

path of the true yogis. A yogi may be able to sit on a bed of nails and more, but his only purpose in doing so is to demonstrate to the unbelieving the power of mind over matter.

Because yogis deal with the prickliest of all subjects—truth—they have always tended to be apart from ordinary society. Many early legends and songs tell of the 'long-haired and wind-girt ones' who are sages and 'see heaven from their homes in the mountains'. In a series of magical chants dating from about 1300 BC there is reference to the 'vratyas', who were probably the forerunners of the modern yogis. They dressed all in black, with a black-and-white ram's hide draped over their shoulders. They cultivated chanting and sat on special seats called 'asandi' while they chanted. Their technical vocabulary was surprisingly "modern" and was taken over almost entirely by the yogis. Their main god was Rudra, god of the wind, who became Shiva. The vratyas inspired the Vishnu devotees who later produced the epic poem of Yoga, the *Bhagavad Gita*.

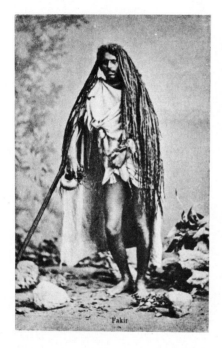

Fakir

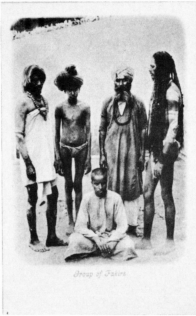

Group of Fakirs

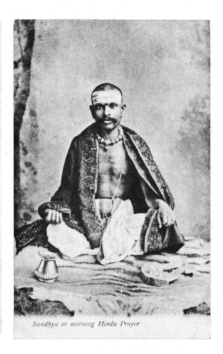

Sandhya or morning Hindu Prayer

A Saint

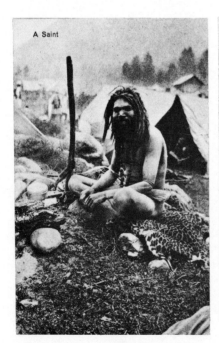

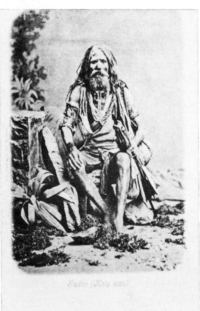

Fakir (Holy man)

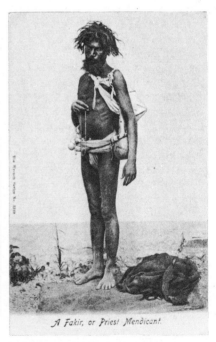

A Fakir, or Priest Mendicant.

Nineteenth-century India abounded in self-appointed saints, street-corner fanatics, and fakirs.
But behind the scenes the true yogis, men of education and learning, were preparing Yoga for its
first great out-going movement.

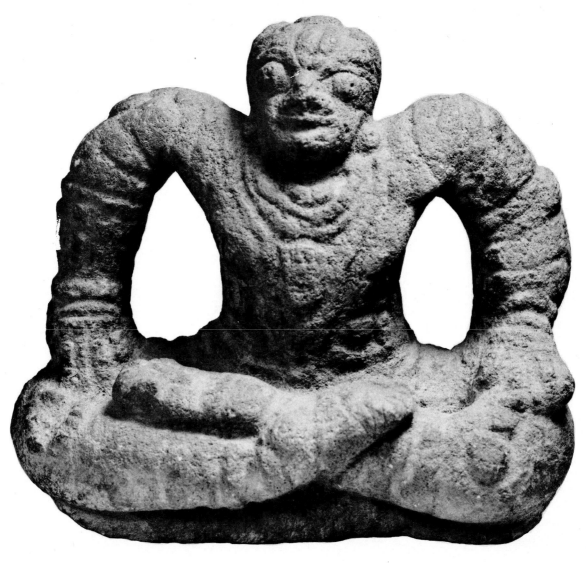

A yogi at his exercises, recorded in a small thirteenth-century stone carving from Madhya Pradesh.

The influence of the yogis was felt all over the Far and Near East. One of Buddha's teachers is thought to have been a master of Yoga, and from the time of Buddha until the early centuries AD Yoga snowballed. Nagarjuna, first great teacher of the Mahayana movement in Buddhism, was a yogi and a magician. Around the fourth century BC, the Yoga sutras of Patanjali were written, and these gave the first text of what forms the basis of most modern Yoga – the eightfold path of Yoga.

Patanjali's work triggered off a whole series of other writings, which in turn stimulated the development of Yoga. The Yogacara school, which formed the basis of Zen Buddhism, was founded, but the techniques of Yoga were being developed mainly through Tantrism. The latter included a belief in the existence of polarity in the body, in the 'kundalini force' which can be made to flow between the two ends of the spine, and in connections between the subtle body and the physical body in the form of 'cakras' and 'nadis'.

From Tantrism developed the body techniques which are now becoming so familiar to the West as Hatha Yoga. This system is unrivalled in its ability to build up the body, but its original purpose was to help withstand the release of kundalini energy,

which, if not properly controlled, can have a devastating effect on the body system.

Yoga works. Nothing which did not work could survive for the three to four thousand years which we are now certain it has existed. It works because it is continually evolving. Although its ultimate concern is with human development at the highest levels, its continual evolution makes it unlike religions, which tend to become fossilized around the sayings of their founders.

A really deep study of Yoga requires time and quiet, so a lot of yogis retired to set up their ashrams in the hills. These little-known retreats had the additional advantage of protecting yogis from being flooded with unwanted and unsuitable students. One of the first requirements of any 'chela' or novice was that he should find his own teacher, and this sometimes involved walking the length and breadth of the Indian continent. Consequently those who were either not enthusiastic or tough enough to withstand the strict traditional training were eliminated before they ever got near to a yogi. Even if the chela found his teacher, his troubles were not over, for the teachers could pick and choose, and put their pupils through immense hardships. The teacher of Milarepa, the Tibetan yogi who lived

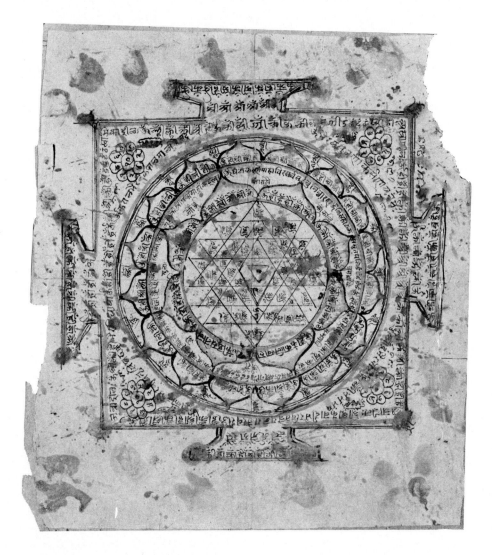

A 'sri yantra' is used as an aid to meditation. This one comes from Rajasthan (*circa* 1800).

about AD 1000, ordered him to build, singlehanded, a ten-storey house in order to work off the bad 'karma'* that he, Milarepa, had accumulated during his early life as a magician.

Yoga continued largely in this pattern with the yogi living in the hills and being sought out by the student until about a hundred years ago. Then the impact of the West began to make itself felt and, conversely, it was also time for Yoga to begin making its impact on the West.

Towards the end of the nineteenth century Ramakrishna, the great yogi philosopher, encouraged his disciple Vivekananda to travel to America and open the door there. In the 1920s Yogananda founded the Self Realisation Fellowship in the United States, where it still flourishes. In India a reformed revolutionary, Aurubindo Ghose, wrote enormous works on the yogic way of life, while a little man of immense compassion called Sai Baba was performing miracles to draw attention to the

need for change. Another giant of the time was Swami Sivananda, who founded the Divine Life Society and began to develop what he called 'Integral Yoga', in which many of the paths of Yoga, such as Bhakti (devotional), Hatha (physical) and Raja (mental), were all united in a working combination. This process has been continuing ever since. Sivananda's ashram was at Rishikesh, a great centre for retreats. His Divine Life Society has produced an enormous number of the present-day international Yoga teachers.

In spite of this progress, Yoga remained for some time under its cloud of non-respectability and it fell to the West and the Western world to recognize the immense effect that Yoga can have on any society. Yoga suffers from the fact that it is very difficult, if not impossible, to study it objectively, from the outside. In order to understand some of the unusual effects of Yoga, you really have to experience them, otherwise they sound too fantastic to believe.

It remained for two eminent Englishmen to study Yoga from the inside. Both of them practised Yoga in depth before they produced books which had a profound effect on Western attitudes. The first of these men was a High Court judge, Sir John

*Karma is the law of cause and effect. Evil acts rebound with evil on the doer, whereas good acts will bring good to the doer. If you kick your neighbour he will come to dislike you. If you honour your neighbour he will come to honour you. Bad karma has to be worked off or paid for before you can move to the next phase of development.

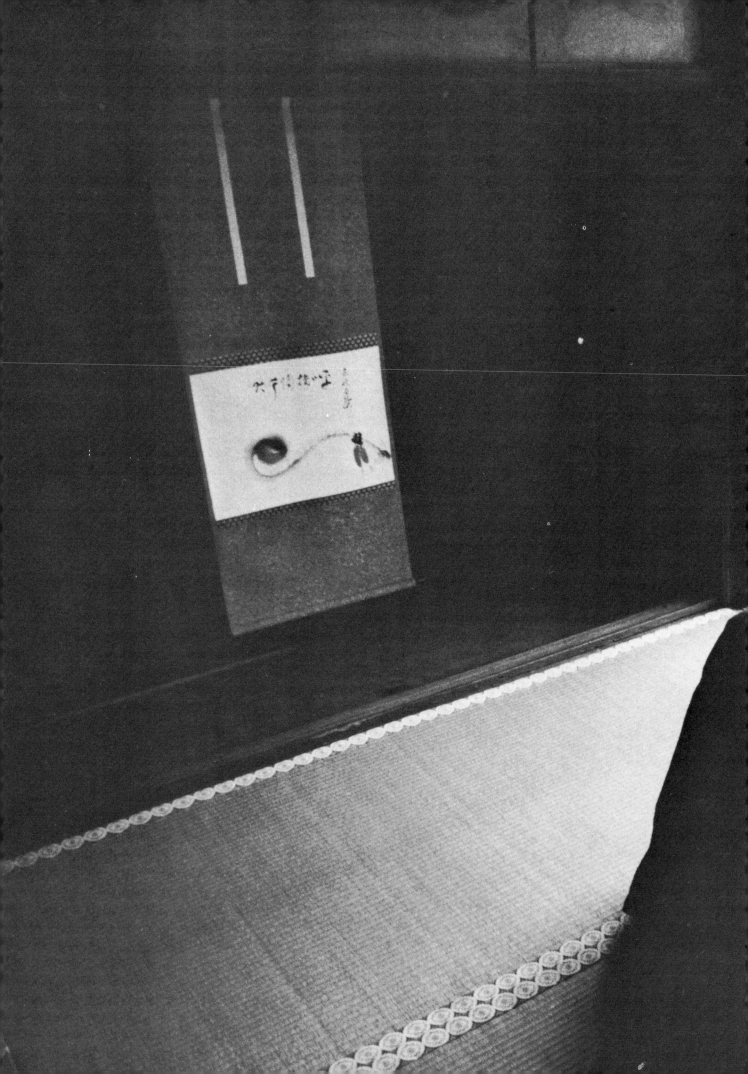

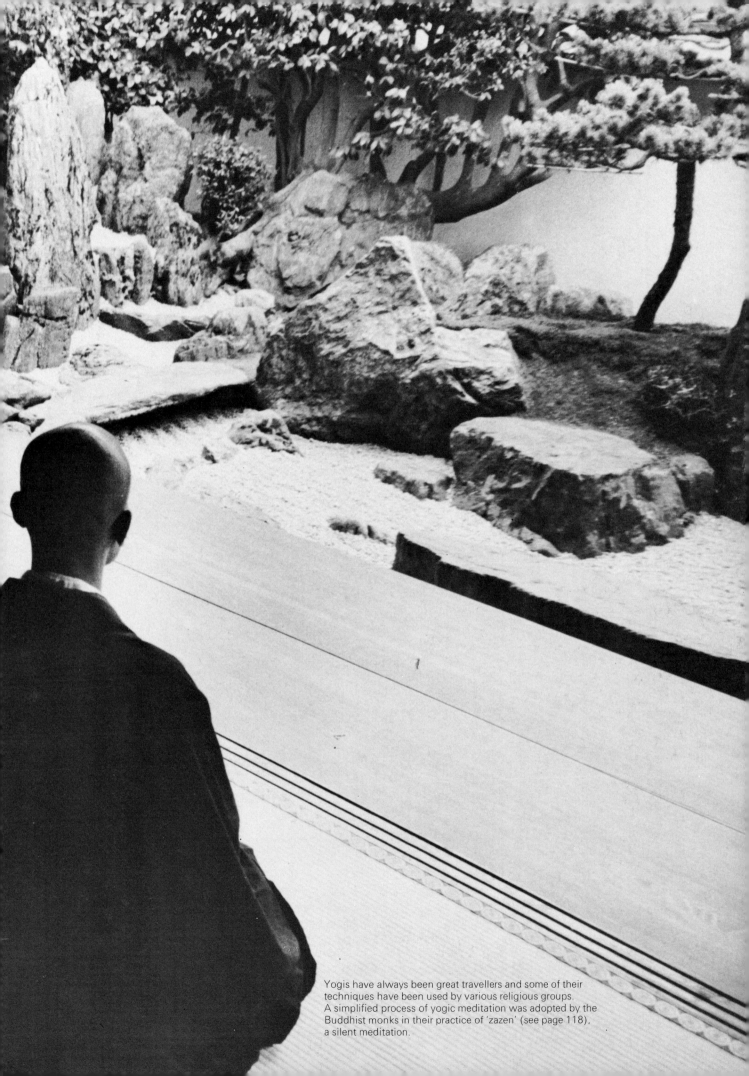

Yogis have always been great travellers and some of their techniques have been used by various religious groups. A simplified process of yogic meditation was adopted by the Buddhist monks in their practice of 'zazen' (see page 118), a silent meditation.

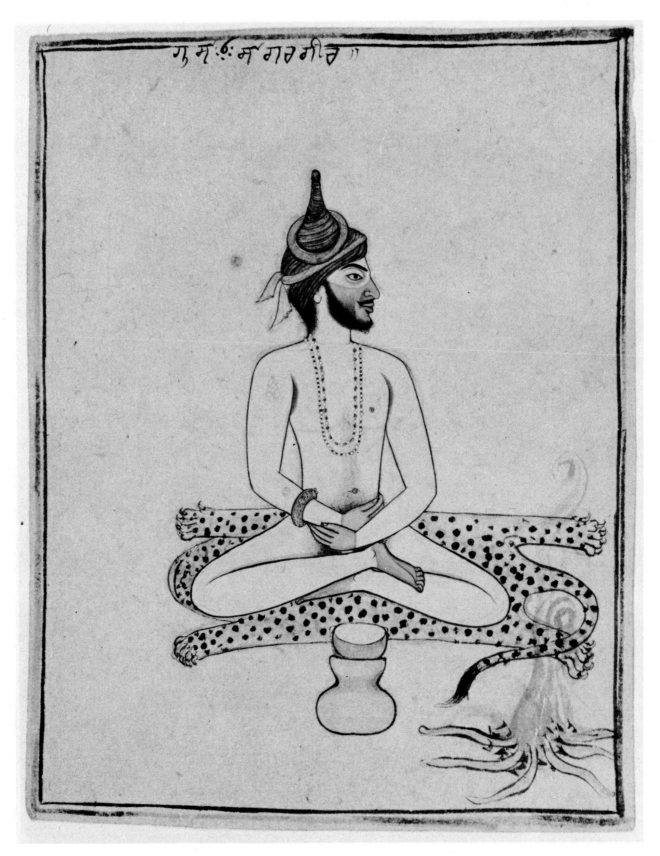

Woodroffe, who wrote under the pen name of Arthur Avalon. His book, *The Serpent Power,* dealt with the technique of Kundalini Yoga and the release of this remarkable force. The second man was Professor Evans-Wentz of Oxford University, who lived among yogis in Tibet for about twelve years and eventually became a yogi himself. He produced many books, among them his famous *Tibetan Book of the Dead,* which describes various techniques for creating transcendental consciousness without the use of drugs. This book was later used by Dr Tim Leary as a guide to the superconscious states which he felt were being achieved through LSD. It is important to note though that yogis have traditionally never recommended the use of drugs for achieving superconscious states: they

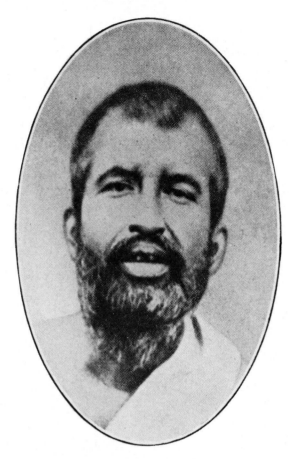

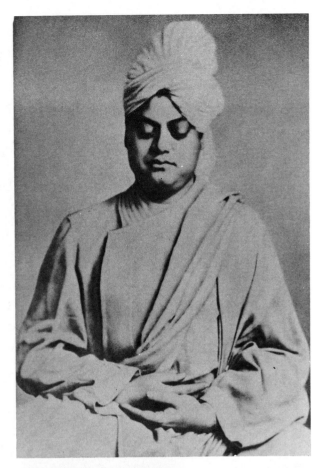

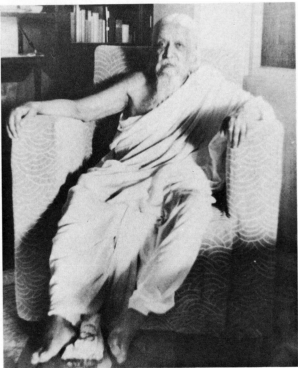

Opposite: An eighteenth-century yogi, a gouache from Mankot.   Above: Ramakrishna, a rural saint.
Right, top and bottom: Vivekananda and Aurubindo, nineteenth-century yogi intellectuals.

believe that they are wholly unnecessary, if not an actual handicap.

Although Vivekananda had immense effect in the West, he was an Indian and consequently to some people slightly suspect as a source of information. However, Professor Evans-Wentz and Sir John Woodroffe were both men of impeccable character and the highest possible standing in their fields in the Western world. From this point on, Yoga had to be taken seriously.

One effect of this more responsible approach is that Yoga has come under scrutiny in research laboratories, and so far has emerged with flying colours. It was at Lonavla in Bombay that one of the first research stations was established, and here the ability of some adepts to control their heartbeats or swallow incredible quantities of poison without any effect was confirmed. More research was carried out on yogis in the West, especially at the Karolinska Hospital in Stockholm, where it became clear that the remarkable legends of yogic control over mind and body were no legend, but solid fact.

A very important investigation was recently carried out in the United States. It was important because the people tested were not adept yogis who had spent a lifetime perfecting their techniques, but Western students who had been practising the technique of transcendental meditation in some cases for only a few months. The results showed quite clearly that the transcendental meditation technique of the much-maligned Maharishi Mahesh Yogi has a beneficial effect on the body chemistry

in that it appears to counteract the effects of stress. It could hardly be possible to give the Western world a greater gift.

Yoga is still evolving. Until very recently it has been confined to a select elite who could insulate themselves from contact with life for years on end. Now it is taking on a form which allows it to blend with Western daily life, thus becoming available to

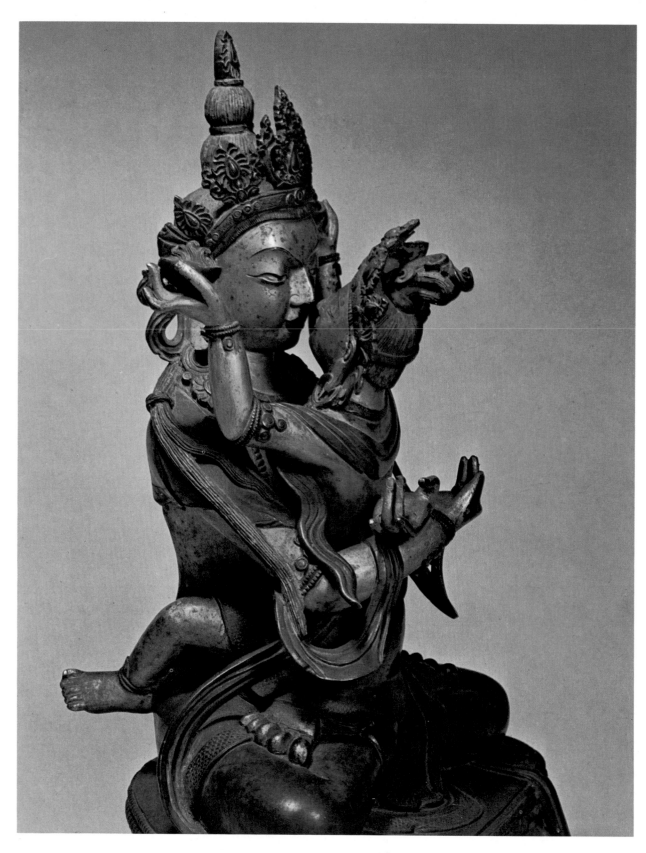

Above: Tantric Yoga has been heavily criticized for its sex
rituals, but much of its thinking underlies other forms of Yoga.
Tantra insists on the existence of polarity in the cosmos,
i.e. a negative cannot exist without there being a positive, or
male without female. Hence in Tantric art a god would always
be shown to be in union with his 'shakti', or female
counterpart, as in this sixteenth-century statuette of
Vajrasattva in union with Supreme Wisdom, Visvatara.

Opposite: A miniature showing a yogi with a pilgrim chela who
is using a band to ease himself in a new posture (*circa* 1640).
The pilgrim's crutch helps to control breathing by putting
pressure on nerve channels in the armpit. It is a yogic accessory;
he is not lame.

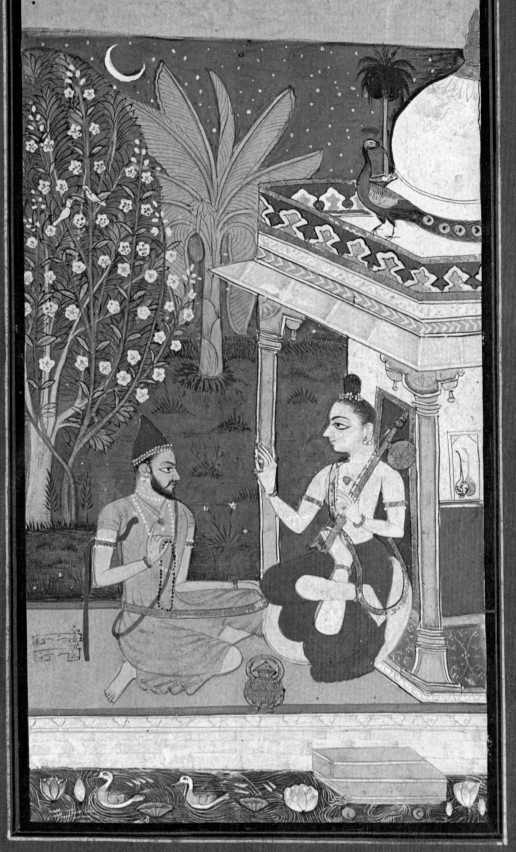

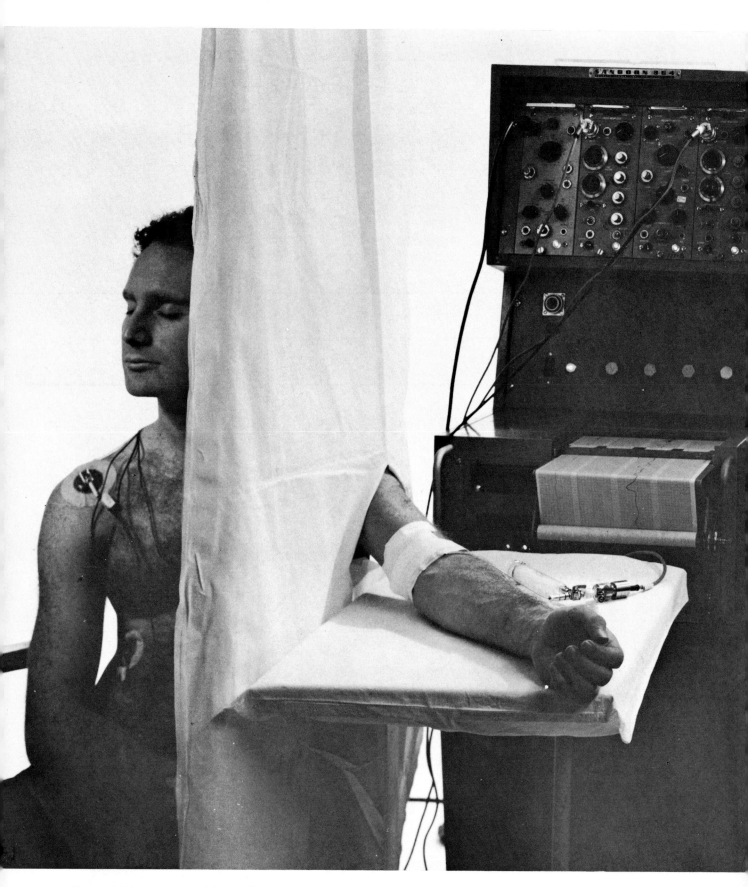

Yoga techniques are successfully standing up to research. At the University of California, meditational techniques were shown to effect positive and beneficial changes in the body chemistry. Here, a subject is screened from the research apparatus so that his observations do not affect his reactions.

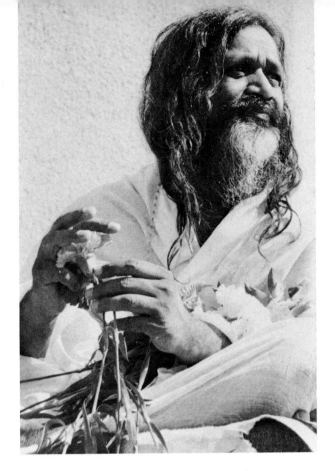

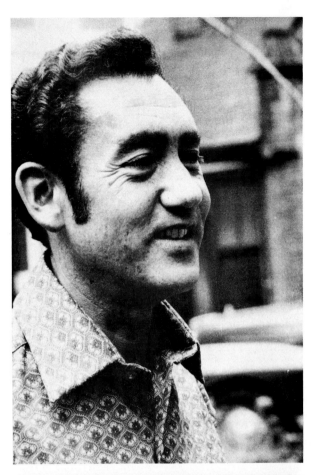

Above: the Maharishi Mahesh Yogi moved into the pop-star scene to create an enormous following. Right, top: Richard Hittleman, TV guru, has reached millions of people.
Right, bottom: B.K.S. Iyengar, master Hatha Yoga technician.

people who can devote only a small period of time to it. It is a process of eliminating some of the time-consuming practices which had previously been considered indispensable. Just as the rishis of the nineteenth century had hoped, the Western laboratories are showing what is essential and what is not.

Books about Yoga now abound, but it is in the new medium of television that the biggest impact has taken place. Yoga is more easily taught by demonstration than by reading and an American yogi, Richard Hittleman, has brought into the Yoga orbit more people than have ever been reached before. To some purists his emphasis is too heavily on the physical, but literally millions of people now know exactly what a Lotus Seat is—even if they will never be able to do it themselves. Yoga is becoming "everyday", instead of strange and rather frightening. It is even becoming respectable. When Yehudi Menuhin, the world-famous violinist, was worn out by the tensions of his long career, it was a yogi, B.K.S. Iyengar, who enabled him to recover his health and with it a new lease of professional life. One might say that this was Yoga's entry into the jet set.

At the present time, followers of Yoga tend to be split into those who want the physical benefits and those who seek the spiritual outlet. The older are more concerned with the waistlines whereas the younger hunger after the spirit. Yoga is not an art, and it is not a religion, yet it can encompass both these things. Yoga is a science.

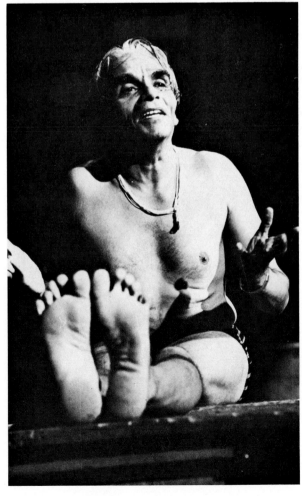

Below: The yogi seen here floating in the River Ganges is not taking an ideal afternoon off—he is performing Plavini Pranayama. In Plavini, the yogi swallows enough air to keep him afloat in the water. His aim is to float weightless so that he is able to reduce any bodily sensations which might disturb his mind and in this way reach a transcendental state more quickly. When he has completed his exercise, he will turn over, belch out the air, and swim to the shore. Experiments with similar weightless conditions have been carried out in Western laboratories and they have shown that the mental effect of such a condition is considerable, but it needs great personal control if it is to be continued for any length of time.

Opposite: Dressed in his usual working garb of a pair of trunks, B.K.S. Iyengar teaches Hatha Yoga in a Central London gymnasium. He is reputed to be an exacting taskmaster and insists on a scrupulously perfect performance of the asanas by his students. Like many yogis, Iyengar now divides his time equally between teaching in India and teaching in the West.

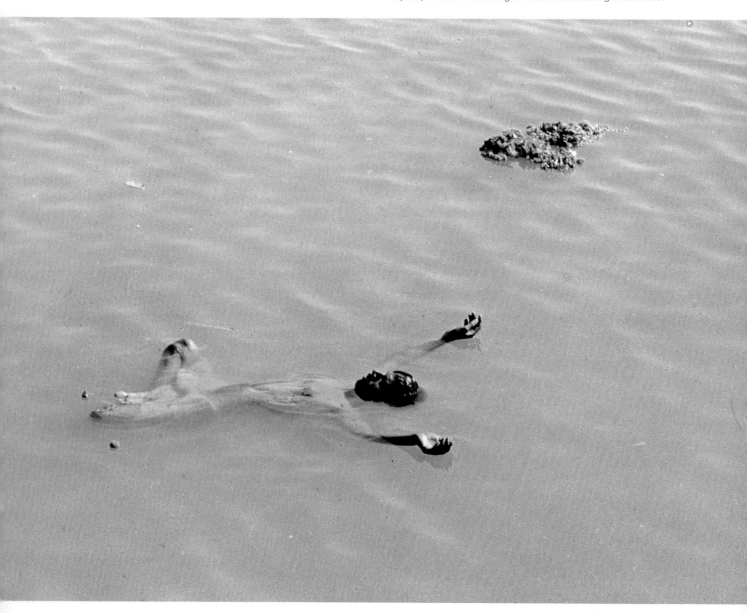

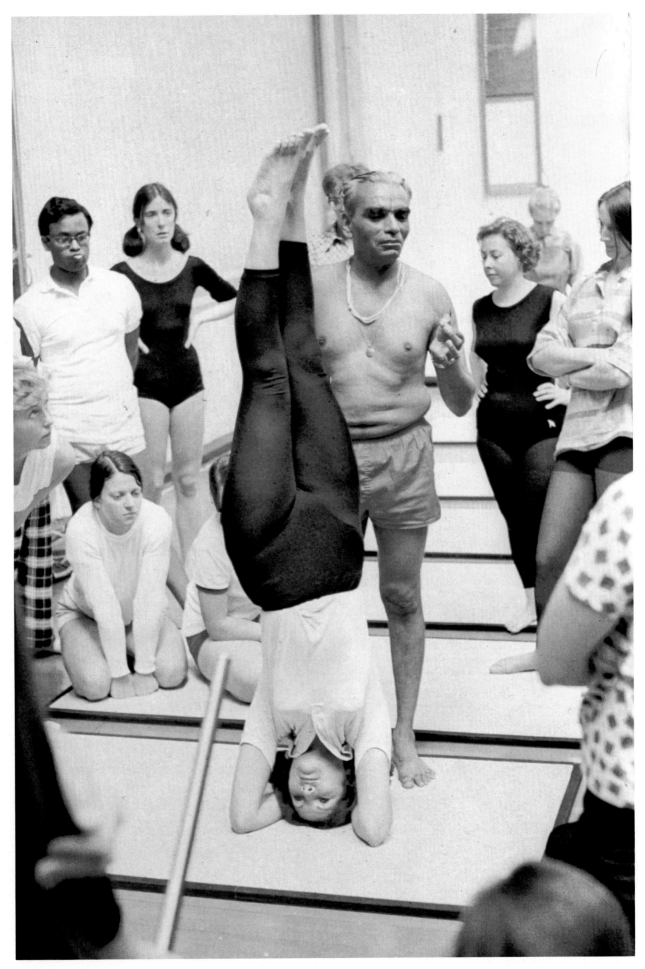

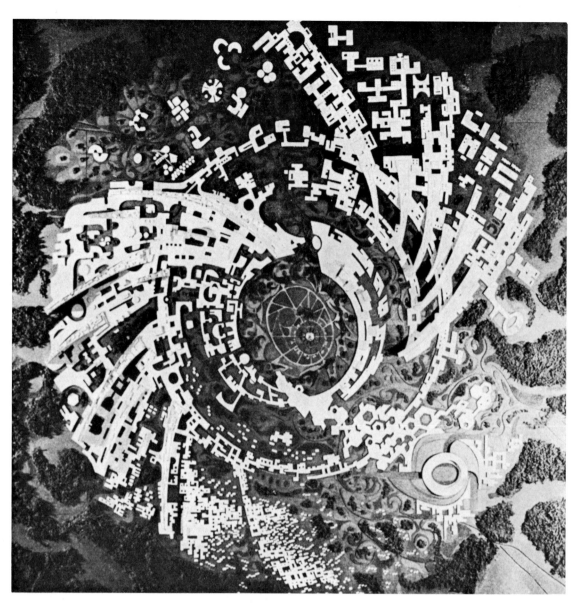

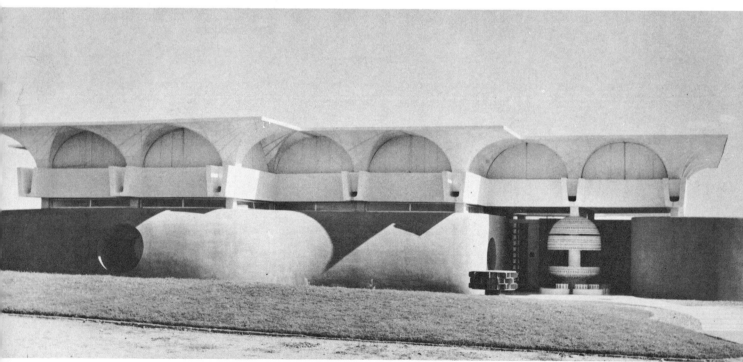

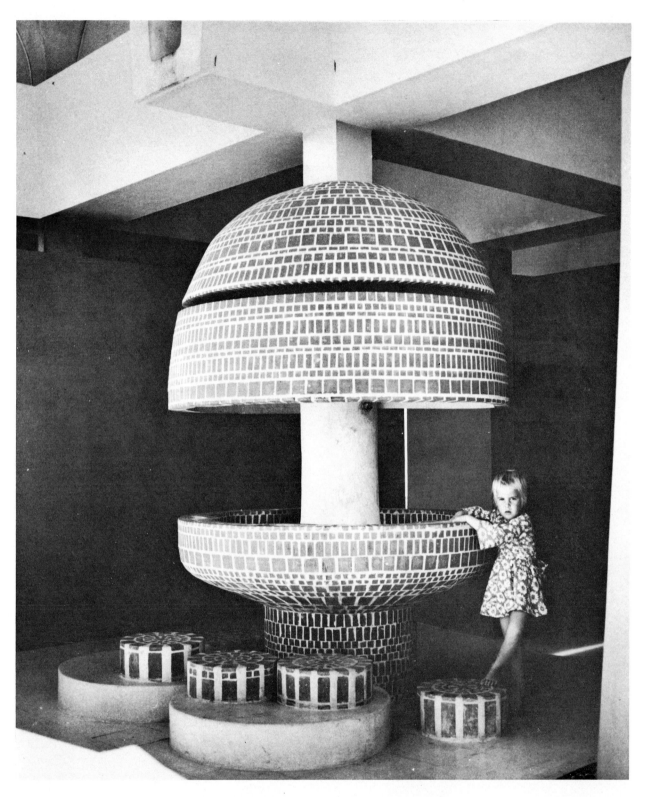

Auroville is one of the show places of India. It is more than just an ashram; it is a whole new town planned on a spiral so that it is capable of indefinite growth. Founded on Yogi Aurobindo Ghose's ideal of the self-supporting organism, Auroville is now run by his descendants.

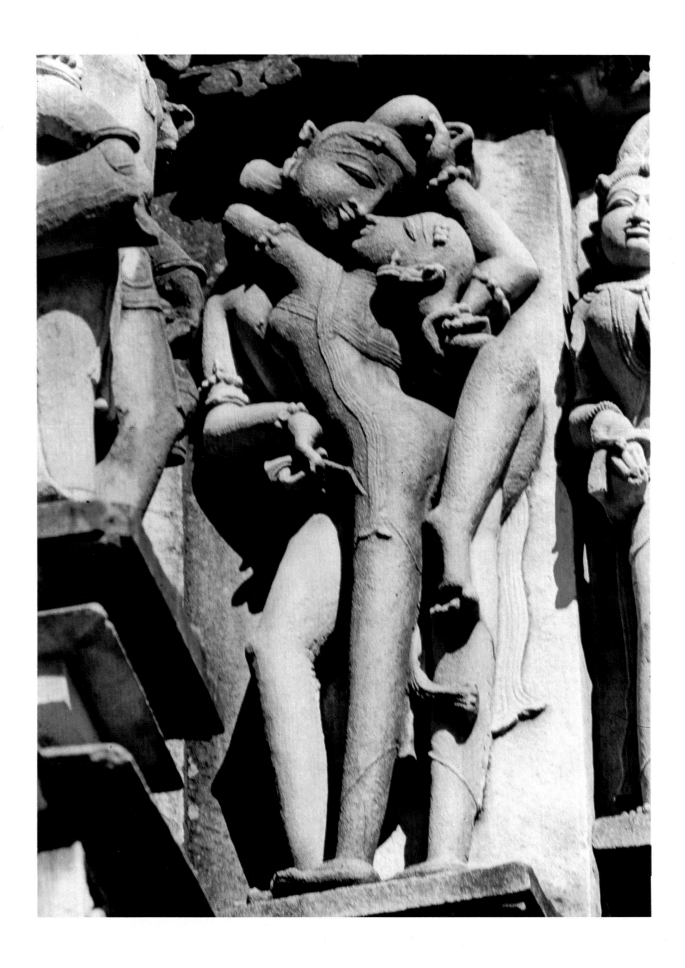

The many erotic statues decorating the facade of the Deva Jagadambi Temple at Khujurao in Madhya Pradesh *(opposite)* demonstrate a joyful acceptance of sex. Contrast this with the Christian myth of Adam and Eve, here interpreted by Lucas Cranach the Elder, where there is a clear attempt to obliterate sex. This may have been a reaction to the Roman sexual orgies, but the result has been a disaster. Any attempt to ignore the human sex dynamic creates a foundation for mass mental illness and dehumanization.

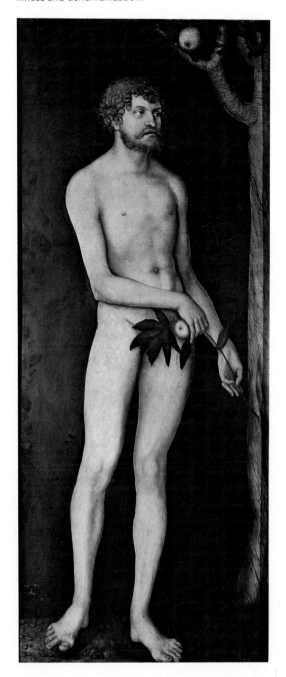 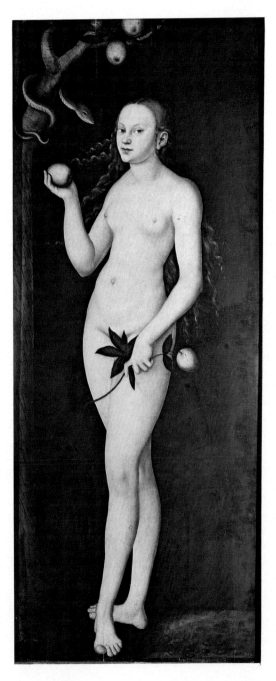

The Legacy of the rishis

and the gurus who can give you the key

All 'rishis', or wise ones, say that you can divide the human race into those who are "awake" and those who are "asleep". Those who are awake have become conscious of the underlying meanings of life, whereas those who are asleep are unaware of anything more than their day-to-day lives. The sleepwalkers tend to live by what is sometimes known as the "hog-in-trough" principle. They think no further than their next pleasure and they are scrabbling all the time for more. Consequently they can be led by the unscrupulous all the way to the slaughterhouse–whether the killing be on the stock exchange or on a battlefield.

Yoga is a way of waking up to the real potentials in this life. Most modern psychologists would agree with the yogis that the average person lives far below his potential abilities, the only difference being that the yogis consider the human potential to be even higher than psychologists generally admit.

There exists within you a treasure house of personal potential to which Yoga is the key.

Because there are many varieties of people there are many forms of Yoga. The Yoga which will suit one person may be wholly unpalatable to someone else. Bhakti Yoga, which is the Yoga of prayers, long meditations and total devotion, is certainly not for everyone. Not only would it be out of character for many, but it would be wholly impractical while running a job and a family. Karma Yoga, the Yoga of good living, is more suited to the Western way of life.

There is no doubt that any system of personal development such as Yoga is better learned from a teacher or 'guru'–if you can find a good one. A guru is less of an instructor in the Western sense than a guide or a setter of example. A true guru is a remarkable person: someone who is sufficiently developed to be able to teach you about yourself both in this world and beyond. Nor surprisingly, true gurus are rare, though they can be found, and the sign of a genuinely high being is that although he owns little or nothing he will want for nothing.

To know exactly what it is like to meet your own guru, read the accounts given by Dr Richard Alpert or Dr Paul Brunton. In his book *Be Here Now*, Dr Alpert says of the moment when he realized that the man he had been brought to see could read every thought that went on in his mind:

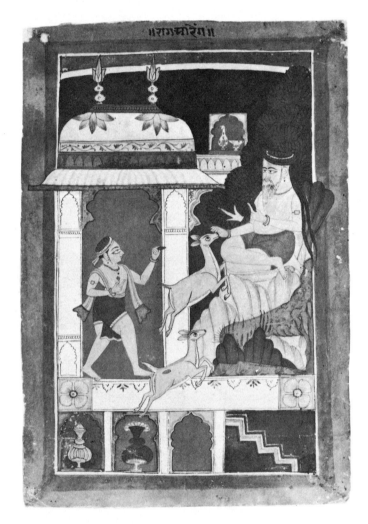

A yogi with his chela and a leaping deer, an illustration to the Indian Musical Mode, Marwar (*circa* 1680).

'And at the same moment, I felt this extremely violent pain in my chest and a tremendous wrenching feeling. And I started to cry. And I cried and I cried. And I wasn't happy and I wasn't sad. It was not that sort of crying. The only thing I could say was that I felt like I was home. Like the journey was over. Like I had finished.'

In fact the journey was only beginning because Yoga is a process of learning and development, but Dr Alpert was home all right.

There is a saying in Yoga that when the chela is ready, the teacher appears. And so it is. You will learn what you are ready to learn. If all that you are ready to know is contained in this book, then that is what you will learn. If part of the book is at the moment too far ahead for you, then although you may read it, it will just not register with you; but maybe if you read it again in six months' time it will hit you so hard that you will say to yourself, 'How in the name of all common sense could I not have realized that before?'

Everyone has a guru somewhere. Every effort you make to find knowledge acts like a voice calling to your teacher's consciousness. Your guru may be thousands of miles away when your plea for knowledge goes up, but, if you are ready, then in ways which you will only later recognize, the knowledge of what to do, where to go, whom to see will come to you. Make no mistake though, gurus are not necessarily hidden in caves in the Himalayas. The physical residence of your guru may be only half a block away from you, but spiritually he can be anywhere and so it is not necessary for you to meet him physically. But should this happen and you do meet him, then, as Richard Alpert says, it is something you will not forget for the rest of your life.

So what, you may ask, is the point of reading a book like this? Well, it can get you through some of the ABC of Yoga so that you will at least know what can happen to you and you can begin to progress on your own. All you need to do is to start trying. The moment you tap into the cosmos and say in all humility 'I need help', someone will surely listen. Under no circumstances though, must you expect someone else to do the work for you. Listen to the words of Chinmoy Ghose, who holds meditation sessions at the United Nations:

'I enter into my disciples and I say, "Look! Here is a box, here is a key, and I am showing you how to open your box. Here is your treasure, it is *your* treasure—not *my* treasure. I show them their own box.... It's the same as with money. When someone works hard and earns money, then he gets more happiness than if someone gives him money. He can say, "I did it, I did it." '

That is all you get out of a guru—the key, the box, and the know-how. You have to open up the box for yourself.

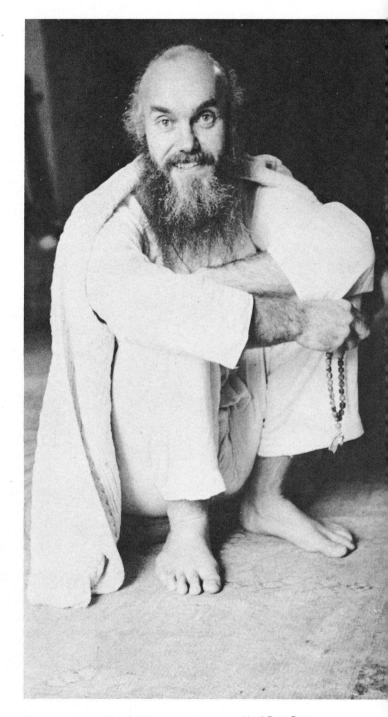

Former professor Richard Alpert, now known as Yogi Ram Dass.

29

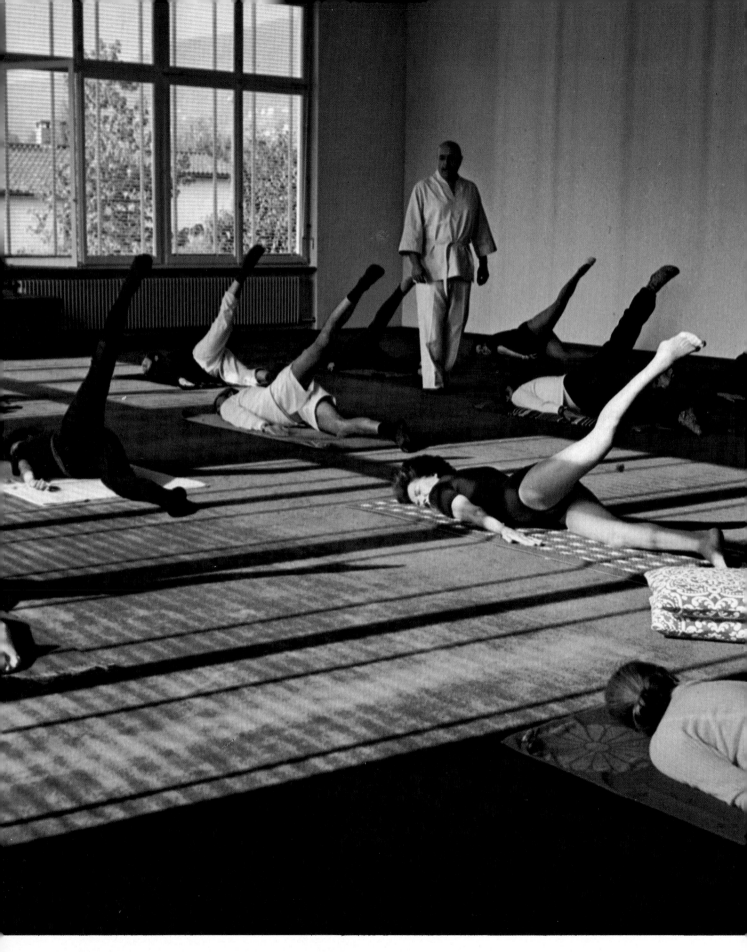

Above: A class at the International Yoga Centre at Caslano in Switzerland. Built by Yogi Robert Walser, the centre was the first European purpose-built Yoga school. The central heating is one concession to the European climate.

Opposite: The yogi depicted in this painting presented by an Indian prince to his wife in 1641 had no problems about keeping warm.

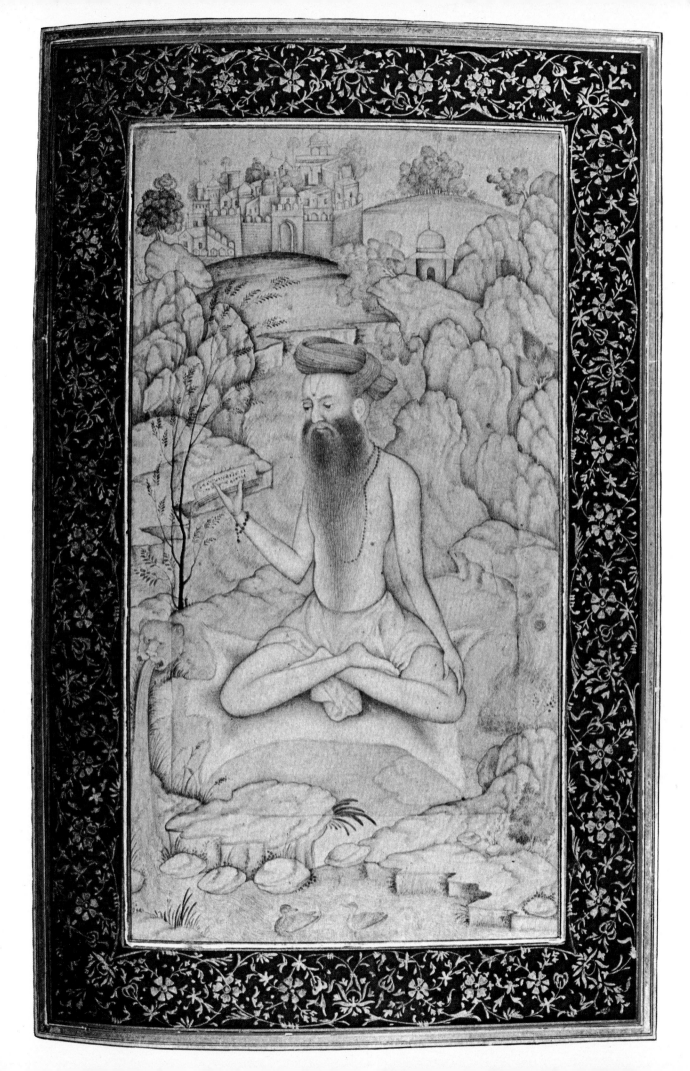

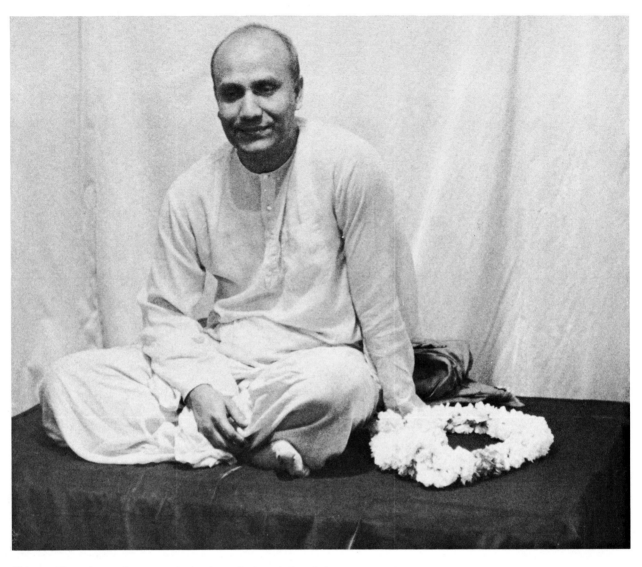

Chinmoy Ghose is a modern guru who teaches only through the mind.

So how do you select a guru? Once again we can turn to the words of Chinmoy. 'Ideally,' says Chinmoy, 'you should be able to tell instantly. You would know if that particular person filled you with utmost joy.' Rather as it was in the case of Dr Alpert. But Yoga teachers of that calibre are rare and perhaps you are not yet sufficiently tuned in. What then? Chinmoy again supplies an answer which brings the whole thing back to earth:

'Do not accept a master just because you have seen the face of a master. You must know what you want, and you can apply the rules just the same to me as to any other spiritual teacher. You simply mark your would-be guru with so many marks out of a hundred.'

To some people this would seem unthinkable. It is rather like checking up to see whether your local bishop is good enough for the job. But then this active, questioning attitude is at the heart of Yoga. You want a guru and you are not too sure. Very well, go ahead and choose him, but do it *using your brain*. You look at him and ask yourself questions. Does he seem honest? Would you trust him always to tell you the truth, and so on, and so on. As Chinmoy Ghose says:

'You mark him so much out of a hundred. If, when you have asked all your questions of yourself, you find that you have only given him thirty out of a hundred, then he is not likely to be for you, no matter how big or famous he may be. But if he gets eighty or ninety out of a hundred, then you have a good chance that he is right for you. You may be told that here is such and such a man who is a great spiritual master, but if you are running to him without using your mind first, then you are mistaken. You must look deep within yourself first. It is the quality [of his disciples] not the quantity that counts.'

In spite of its concern with the spiritual, Yoga is not a religion. It is no hocus-pocus and hey-hey Lawdy-Lawdy!, claiming that all will be given to you if you just believe (and place a suitable donation in the collecting box, please!). Yoga will never shower you with gifts and promises. Yoga, in fact, is just about the epitome of the adage that 'God helps those who help themselves'.

32

ANYONE CAN BE A YOGI

In his book *Light on Yoga*, the famous Yoga teacher B.K.S. Iyengar defines a yogi as 'anyone who follows the path of Yoga'. The very minute that you begin your first study of Yoga, you become a yogi – for have you not already begun to 'follow the path of Yoga'?

You can learn Yoga any time, all the time. Yoga goes with you everywhere. It can be in the way you walk, the way you talk to people, the way you eat. You do not achieve it, you live it. All the time you live like a yogi, you are a yogi. When you do not live like a yogi, you cease to be a yogi. Hundreds and thousands of people have found that by starting with a few very simple body exercises, they have eventually finished up changing their whole lives.

The yogis believe that there is virtually no limit to your development if you follow the three paths of:

1. the Asanas (physical exercises and postures),
2. Pranayama (the direction of life force by breathing), and
3. Raja Yoga (the control of the mind).

Western medicine accepts that the mind can influence the body to the extent of creating psychosomatic illnesses, which are actual and not

Even the English climate occasionally allows a traditional Yoga class among the trees.

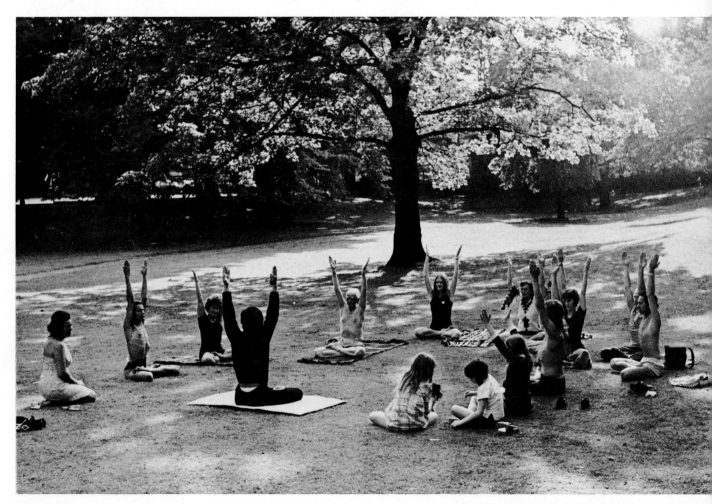

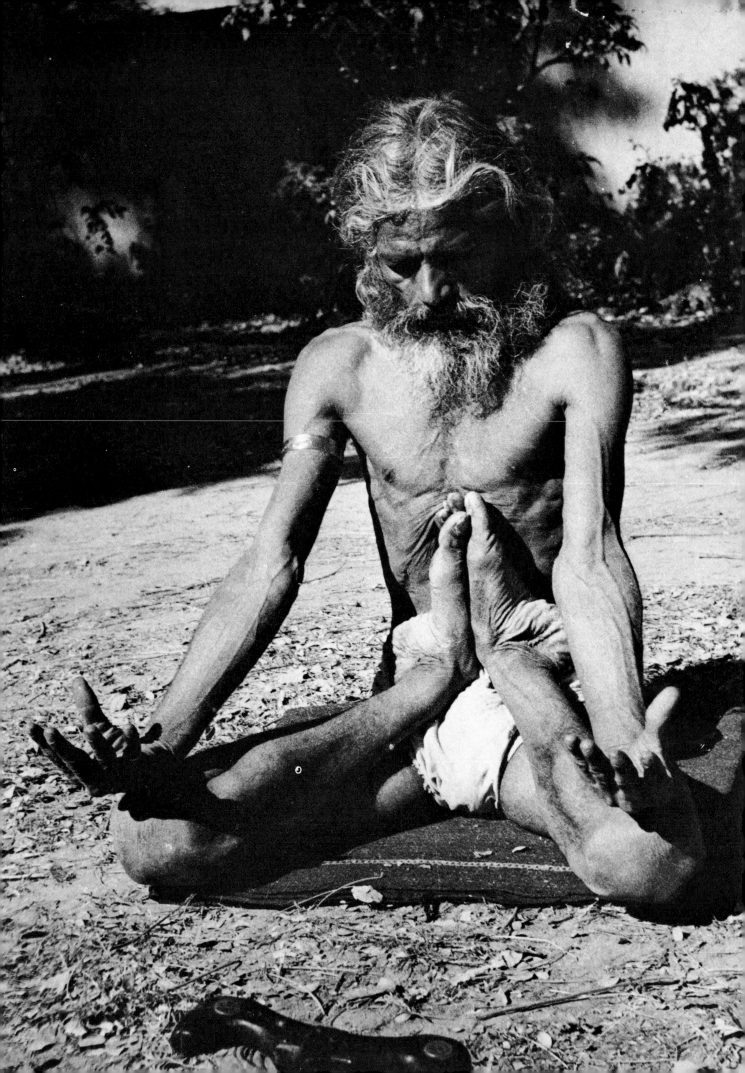

imaginary illnesses, but for some reason it is slow to accept that the process can also work the other way round. The yogis, on the other hand, say that the body and the mind interact, and that your physical actions can alter your mental outlook, as well as the other way around. For this reason every effort is always made to create good health, and this means not just a lack of actual illness, but positive health.

Positive health in turn leads to dynamic control and this can be demonstrated in its more extreme form by the trials which some Tibetan yogis put upon themselves in order to prove the extent of their development. One such trial, called 'tumo', was a process of heat control, and a yogi who could carry it out successfully was known as a 'repa', which means cotton-clad one. The yogi sat in the snow with only a wet sheet wrapped round his body on a dark, icy, winter night at an altitude of about 10,000 feet in the Himalayan mountains. Any average human being would have been quite literally frozen solid in a matter of minutes, but these remarkable men exerted such fantastic control over their life force that they generated enough heat with their bodies to dry the sheet and melt the snow around where they sat. Their success was measured by the size of the circle of melted snow surrounding them. A fully-qualified repa was required to dry three sheets one after the other on his body. The badge of proficiency was a cotton gown, the repa's only garment even in the sub-zero temperatures of the Tibetan mountains. His control over his body temperature was so complete that he needed no other clothing.

What is it about Yoga that makes it possible for men to perform feats which would be quite impossible to ordinary human beings? The answer may well lie in the integrating effect which Yoga has on the human organism.

In the West, man has learned to tap cosmic forces mainly by mechanical means. He discovered how to use the power of the petroleum molecule to drive a motor car and how to split the atom. Yet in the same civilization there are people who have so lost control over their minds and bodies that they are forced to take pills to perform the simple, natural act of sleeping.

Moreover, the Western world largely follows the mediaeval Christian idea that a man has only two parts*, a body and a soul, and that the two have no contact with or control over each other. This concept encouraged the hopelessly self-defeating idea that the body is a handicap to living and that the first aim of spiritual advancement should be to ignore the body, treating it as "sinful". The result of any attempt to live in this way is to create a state of internal conflict in the human organism which produces not only a permanent drain of energy, but literally whole populations who are emotionally, mentally and physically distorted. The blood-sodden history of Western wars, tortures, and persecutions shows how true this is.

*This was not part of the original Christian teaching which was much closer to Yoga.

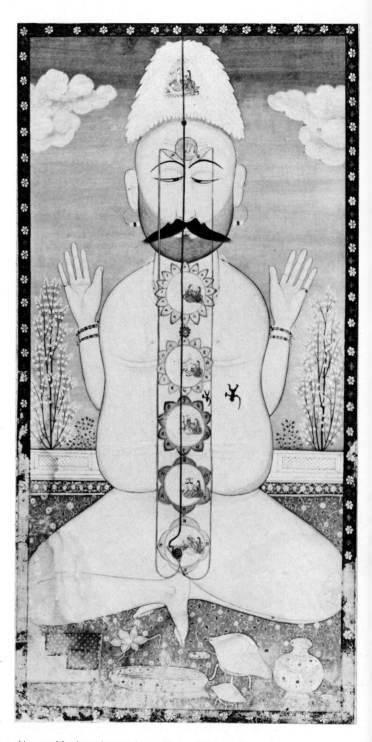

Above: Much ancient and occult knowledge has been preserved through Yoga. The major cakras or wheels—the cosmic force centres of the human organism—are one such example. Their positions, which are shown diagrammatically in this eighteenth-century drawing, are traditionally read from the bottom up. Although the cakras are considered to be a part of the astral body, they have important psycho-physical links and relate in number to the tension sections found by Dr Wilhelm Reich. In physical terms, they correlate roughly with the endocrine system, the stimulation of which contributes to the extraordinary effectiveness of some Yoga practices.
Opposite: A modern yogi, using Kandasana. This has the effect of stimulating the second and third cakras, Svadihasthana and Manipura, which in turn affect the digestion.

Yogis consider that a man has not one body but three, in which are 'sheaths' of increasing density. Roughly speaking the body states are likened to the condition of steam, water, and ice: the soul or spirit being the steam, the subtle or astral body being the water, and the final ice form being the gross or physical body, the everyday shape we move about in on this planet. Herein lies some of the extraordinary effectiveness of Yoga. Unlike the mediaeval Western concept which ignores one part of man and tries to drag the remaining two apart, Yoga is designed to integrate the whole human organism.

Yogis believe that there are power points, 'cakras', and power channels, 'nadis', in the subtle body which are linked closely to those of the physical body. There are generally considered to be seven main cakras, which coincide roughly with the main parts of the endocrine system but which are positioned at points in the spine. Minor differences exist in the detail of exactly where the cakras are positioned, some schools of thought preferring to consider only six cakras whereas others work with eight. However, the main principles remain unaltered. The bottom cakra, the 'muladhara' cakra, lies at the base of the spine and the top one, the 'sahasrara' cakra, is at the crown of the head, where a monk has his tonsure or a Turk his top-knot. Joining the cakras is a nadi called 'sushuma'. There are also two nadis known as 'ida' and 'pingala', which correspond to the sympathetic cords in the physical body.

One of the fundamental aims in Yoga is the controlled release of what is called the 'kundalini' power, which flows between the base of the spine and the crown cakra. An uncontrolled release can be dangerous, rather like a short circuit. The whole organism has to be conditioned to take the extra load, which is only released very gradually from one cakra to the next.

Did the orthodox medical world but realize it, their own emblem of the winged staff with two entwined snakes is nothing more than a symbolic representation of what the yogis consider to be the power channels of the subtle body. The straight staff is sushuma, ida and pingala are the entwined snakes, and the points at which they cross correspond roughly to the positions of the intermediate cakras. The wings at the top of the staff? It is easy to see how they have been modified from the thousand-petal lotus symbol which is traditionally used for sahasrara. This symbol adopted by healers is extraordinarily appropriate since basically it is a diagram of the power centres of the human organism. Control these and you have gained control over the entire organism.

Because of the care that yogis bestow on their bodies, superficial observers tend to assume that Yoga is nothing more than a somewhat unusual form of physical culture, typified by the Lotus Seat and standing on one's head. But in Yoga the real you is not considered to be the physical body alone. Your body is like a suit of clothes that is worn, looked after until it is worn out, and then eventually exchanged for another—for the yogis believe in re-incarnation.

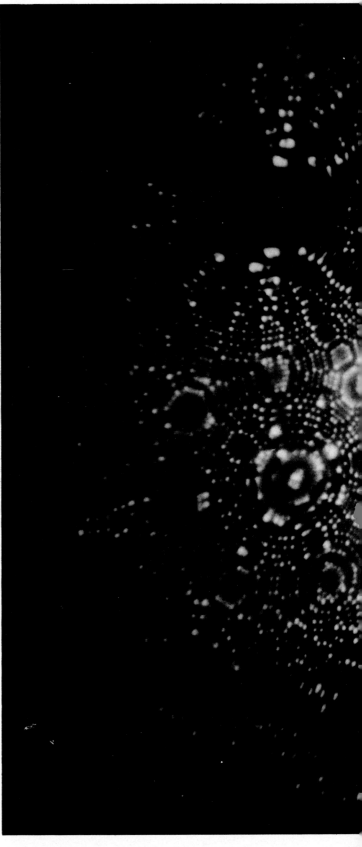

You need not accept any of this to practise Yoga because Yoga is not a religion. It is not necessary to believe in any set of dogmas. The yogis say, 'Believe nothing that you cannot or do not experience for yourself.'

Maybe this all seems to be getting a bit far out, but it is an interesting fact that the latest scientific

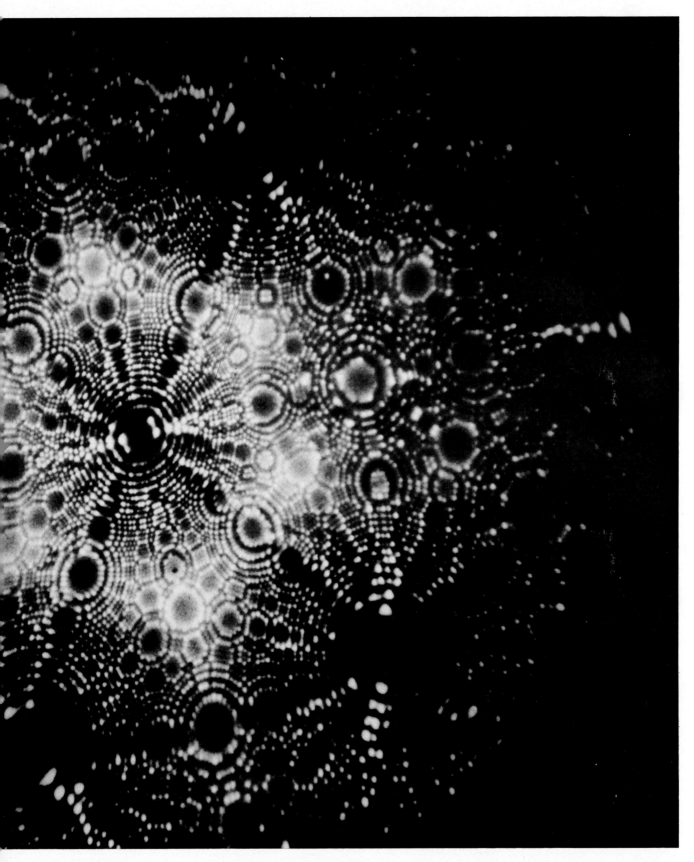

experiments on the structure of life are tending to confirm yogic thoughts which pre-date them by thousands of years.

Yoga works, and every research laboratory will confirm it.

Helium field ion micrograph of a tungsten point. The further science goes into the structure of the cosmos, the more the statements of the early yogis seem to be confirmed. They have long claimed that all matter was ultimately made up of vibrations and that only the scale of vibrations caused flesh to differ from stone.

The eightfold path of yoga

The emphasis put on any part of Yoga has always been a matter of individual choice, but for nearly a thousand years Yoga has generally been thought to consist of eight 'paths' or 'limbs'. It was this form which was the first to be set down, by Patanjali in the fourth century BC.

Times change and so does Yoga. It is a continually developing system and great confusion arises from the varying uses that have been made of the words which describe the paths of Yoga. It is likely that as Western scientific research digs deeper into Yoga the present eight steps will be changed slightly but they, or something like them, will inevitably form the foundation for the study of Yoga for some time to come. They are as follows:

1. yamas
The first steps in mind control, entailing the attempt to live positively through the virtues of simple cleanliness, honesty (to self as well as others) and respect toward all men.
2. niyamas
Those things which it is positively directed a yogi should avoid, such as lying, stealing, greed, killing and any form of excess.
3. asanas
The learning and practice of the postures for physical/mental development.
4. pranayama
The control of the life force, by means of systematic breathing.
5. pratyahara
The ability to withdraw and lose contact with the outer world as a step toward Dharana.
6. dharana
The concentration of thought on any point either inside or outside the body.
7. dhyana
The intensification of concentration until the mind is wholly absorbed by the object.
8. samadhi
For lack of a better word, this is best described as superconsciousness. The exact sensations will vary from person to person and obviously it is not possible to explain a mindless superconsciousness in the words of ordinary consciousness. But in fact many people achieve samadhi in flashes during their life and especially in childhood. Thinking back over your life, no matter how generally unhappy you may

have been, you will be able to recall short periods of maybe only minutes or even seconds when you experienced an immense joy and a sense that everything was completely right with the world. You may have realized the beauty of water, the logic of mathematics or simply the fact that it is quite right for babies to make noises at both ends.

There are two main forms of samadhi. They are very different, but each will produce a sense of bliss. In the first, 'kalpa samadhi', the bliss is only temporary; like the LSD trip, it comes to an end, and one returns to one's grumpy old self. Possibly grumpier, because of the vision one has had to leave behind.

The second form of samadhi is an entirely transcendental state which in effect is a complete reconditioning of the mind. Old ideas are sloughed off like an unneeded suit of clothes, and a new person emerges, a person whose view of life and methods of living can never be the same again. This is 'nirvi kalpa samadhi'.

The steps are numbered consecutively, but this does not mean that the process is consecutive and that you cannot begin number two until you have completed number one. On the contrary, you can move forward on all paths at the same time even though not necessarily at the same pace. It is admittedly a lot easier to achieve a good standard in the asanas than to arrive at samadhi, but the one helps the other.

No path can be wholly separated from the others and they all interact so that movement along any path will reflect some benefit in the others. The first five paths tend to look outward, whereas the last three tend to look inward. Body and mind interact but it is the mind which is the senior partner.

hOW NOT TO crIpple yOURSELF DOING YOGA

During the wintertime you can often see sun-tanned people limping around ski resorts on crutches or with their arms in slings. These are the part-time holiday skiers. There is nothing wrong with skiing as a sport but your body does have to be in the right condition for it. You have to go slowly down the beginners' slopes before you can charge down a slalom run, or you find yourself in trouble.

Much the same thing applies to Yoga. Yoga is not dangerous. The only way you can get into trouble is if you break all the rules and go at it like a bull at a gate.

Because we in the West lead such inactive lives many of the postures are strange and sometimes a little difficult at first. It is even difficult for most of us to learn how to sit on the ground instead of in a chair. That graceful posture the Lotus Seat is one of the most envied positions in Western eyes and more people have damaged themselves by trying to force their stiffened joints into this position than any other.

Don't do it. Stop competing against the clock. Stop competing against yourself. You get no halo for a rushed virtuoso performance. A few asanas slowly

Beautiful patterns in the snow for the skilled—falls for the unskilled.

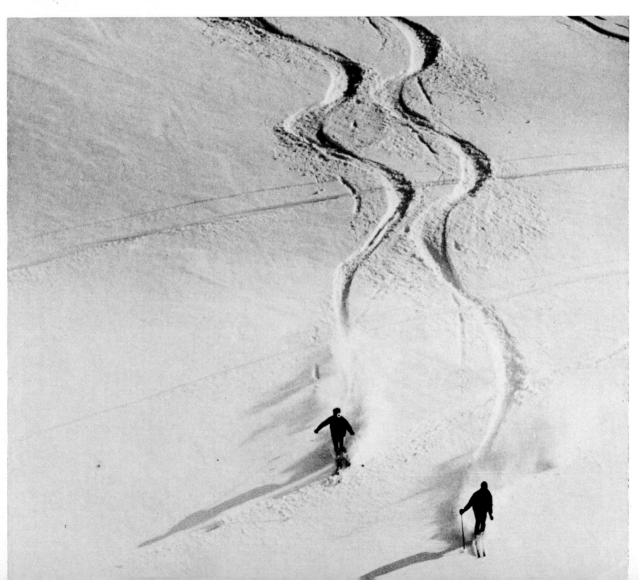

learned and performed gracefully and gently every day will lead you into the Yoga way of life. Trying to be a virtuoso is just an ego trip.

It's that old hog-in-trough business again. 'Look, here is the great ME doing all those difficult complicated Yoga postures. I bet you can't do as many of them as I can!' Ego trips take you nowhere. How can they if everything is centred round you personally?

Nobody is saying that you should not want to improve yourself, that it's wrong to want a better body to live in, a better life. Fine, only don't be greedy about it or rush it. Developing yourself for a new way of life is a gradual, growing process. Watch any living, growing thing, a puppy or a plant. The fully-grown developed features do not suddenly attach themselves from the outside; they develop from the inside – and so do we.

Whether you gain benefit or whether you damage yourself by doing Yoga postures depends largely on the state of mind in which you approach them. This is why before anything else chelas are taught an understanding of what is meant by the yamas and niyamas.

It's obvious that these ethical standards will immediately affect your daily session of Yoga postures. If you sit down in a state of personal greed, then you may well strive too hard to achieve the positions. If you extend the precept of non-injury to others, it becomes absurd that you should then injure yourself by abusing the limitations of your own body. You can only do it if you break the rules and go on a mindless ego trip.

Hurting yourself is no virtue. Self-torture is usually a symptom of repressed sex. It is no accident that flagellation and barefoot penitence are found largely amongst religious orders which allow no normal sex life. If you want to hurt yourself, there must be a reason for it and the path of true self-development is to find out why and change.

Self-study of our own bodies has been so badly inhibited by the Western "flesh is sinful" outlook that some people find real trouble in actually becoming sufficiently aware of their bodies to realize whether they are damaging themselves or not. For these people there is only one path to take and that is the path of concentrated, objective body-consciousness.

At one time in life, all of the sensations coming from the body to the brain were equally welcomed and uninhibited. So you are not learning anything new when you take to body consciousness; you are

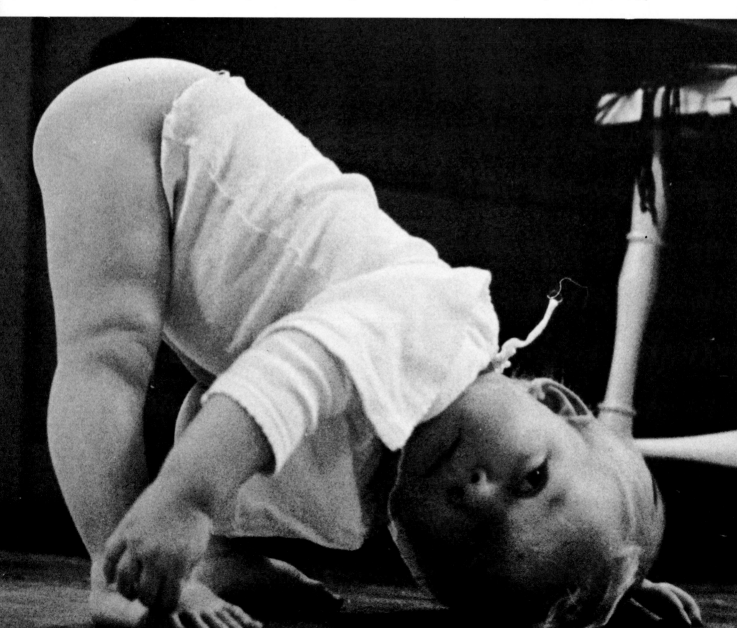

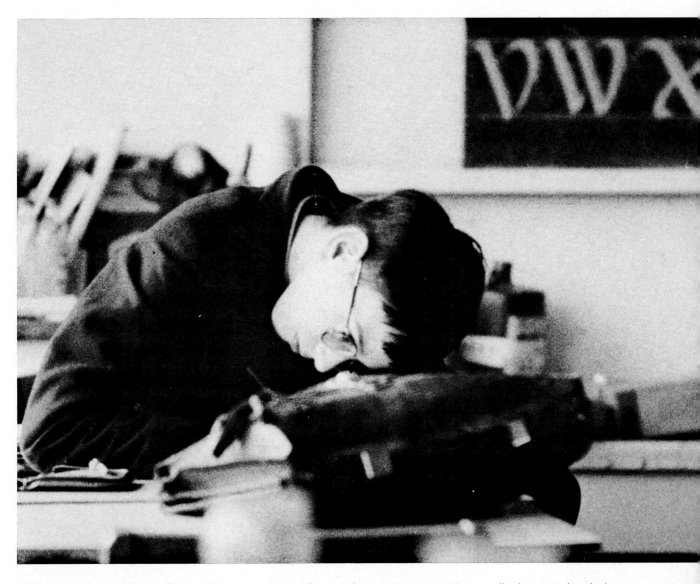

simply re-learning those things which you learned as a very young child.

When you touch something, be it hot water or a piece of silk, messages about what you are feeling are sent up to your brain. These continue to be sent up irrespective of your age. The brain of a young child receives these messages and stores them all up as knowledge; enjoys the pleasurable ones and hates the unpleasant ones. The images are vivid and fresh. Then along comes the "flesh is sinful" conditioning and so what happens? The messages still come up from the fingers or tongue and some of them are inevitably pleasurable. They cannot be shut off at the fingers, but the child has been told that to feel pleasure at the touch of silk is sinful and the touch of flesh is unmentionable. The only way to stop these sensations coming through is to shut off the main reception centre for them. The trouble is that in doing this the whole series of impressions very often gets shut off as well, the unpleasant as well as the pleasant.

So what is wrong with losing unpleasant sensations? Everything, because these are our warning signals. A bad taste can indicate poisonous food. Pain from our skin may mean a burn or a cut, and pain from our joints a strain or a tear.

Infant suppleness can only too easily give way to hunched shoulders and stunted growth if there is no adequate physical training.

People who are on an ego trip or a guilt trip turn off the warning systems in the brain because the messages coming in conflict with the over-riding wish in their minds, whether it be ambition or the desire for punishment. In the first case, the pain warning is cut out because it gets in the way of ambition, and so damage to the body takes place. In the second case, the danger can be even greater because the pain is actually enjoyed. The greater the pain, the greater the inner pleasure because it satisfies the conditioning that pleasure from the flesh is sinful and must therefore be converted into pain, thus becoming "good".

It's an extraordinary mix-up, but it happens. So in Yoga we have to re-educate ourselves to receive and acknowledge *all* of the messages that come in from the body, whether they are painful or pleasurable. Only in this way is our total of experience and awareness expanded.

BODY CONSCIOUSNESS

There is no better route to body consciousness than that which you took as a baby. So, for a start, look at your hands. Hold them out in front of you and examine them carefully. Look at their colour, their texture. Move the fingers as if to grasp something. See how they move and see where the joints are. So far you have been observing your hands from the outside. Now transfer your thought to the *inside* of your body. Repeat the movements of your fingers and hands but this time close your eyes so that you can concentrate on feeling what is happening inside as the muscles work.

Squeeze your hand tight to make a fist and feel which parts of the fist are hard and which are soft. Bend your arms at the elbows and pull your fists up as tight against the shoulders as you can. Feel where the pressures are. Now relax your arms and fix into your mind what a muscle feels like when it relaxes.

Carry this process of re-awakening all the way through your body. Your arms, your legs, your feet. Twist your back. Open your mouth and close it; feel how the jaw works. *Learn to feel your body from the inside.* Accept *all* the information that comes into your brain about what is going on in your body. What you must do is learn to understand its language. Learn to recognize the signals which say you are working it too hard.

In case this seems a lot of fuss just to get to know a frame that you have been living in for the whole of your life, remember that this ability to direct your consciousness to any part of your organism is a fundamental part of Yoga practice and you will be using it every time you practise any one of the postures: sometimes to direct 'prana', the life force, into a particular part of the body, and sometimes to help energize the cosmic power within you and release it gradually through the body.

Many of the physical exercises of Yoga are stretches which are designed to help ease the nervous tension out of your system because when you are tense mentally, you become tense physically. If you are going to stretch the tension out of a muscle, it must be done gently—very gently.

Your muscles have an independent and automatic protective system built into them. Say, for example, you are stretching your back muscle when it is tense. It will not stretch very much, and if you continue the attempt it will tear. Now suppose the same muscle is relaxed. It will stretch to a certain extent.

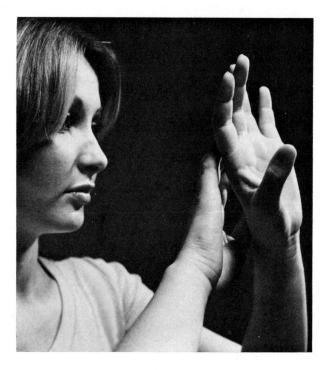

Above: Is this really me? You ask the same questions as you asked when you were a baby *(opposite)*.

But suppose you try to stretch too quickly or too much. The muscle's immediate reflex reaction is to contract in order to try and prevent damage by making itself stronger. Now provided you do not increase the pull at this stage, your muscle will be all right. But if you do increase the pull, you will be doing it when the muscle is in the wrong condition for stretching and so you are more or less bound to damage it. If ever there was a case for making haste slowly, it is in learning the asanas.

One last simple precaution that you should take before starting your course of Yoga postures. Have a medical check-up and tell your doctor what you propose to do. Some medics are now all for Yoga and will bless you as being one more sensible person who is going to be less likely to crowd into his consulting room with illnesses that need never have happened. Other, more old-fashioned, doctors who usually know little about Yoga tend to be a bit doubtful, but it is really only because they are being careful and you cannot blame them for that.

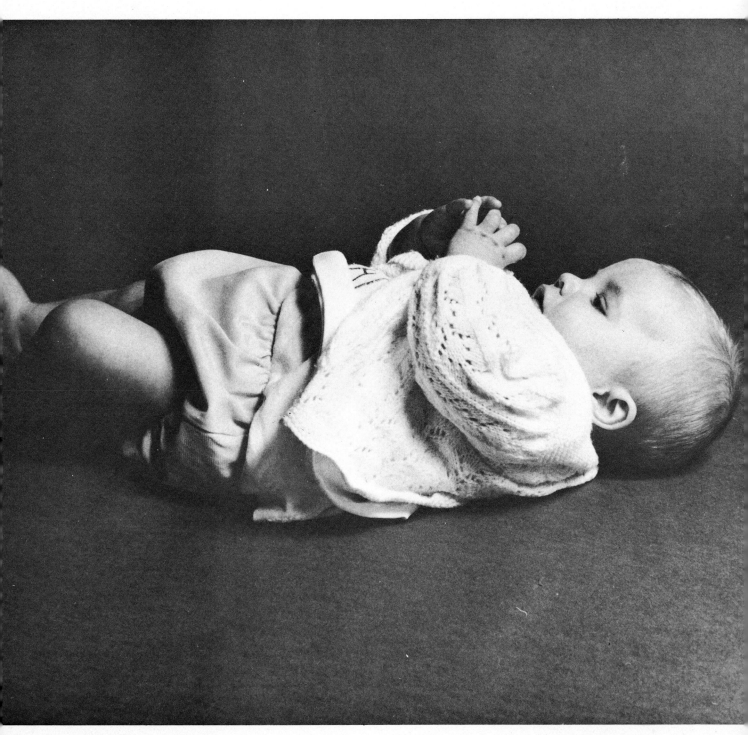

hail, SMILING MORN

or how to get a good night's sleep without pills

Do you wake blithely of a morning to say, 'Good morning, God!' or is it just, 'Good God, morning!'? Let's not pretend we don't know the symptoms, all the way from the legs of lead to the burning eyelids and the parrot-cage mouth.

There is no doubt that if you want to get up fresh in the morning, the only way to do it is to have a good night's sleep. Like so many Yoga techniques, the effect is that of an ascending spiral. In other words, the more you develop your yogic sleeping and waking technique, the more efficient you become and the less and less sleep you need to obtain the same amount of rest.

Many yogis are four-hour-a-night people: they find that this is ample sleep for their normal working day. But once again, don't try to make an end-game out of this. Don't set yourself a target and say, 'In future, the great "I" will only sleep five hours a night.' The chances are that the only thing which will happen is that you will get completely tired out. A reduced sleeping time arrives as a bonus, but only after you have organized proper sleeping techniques for yourself.

Scientists have investigated the nature of sleep, and amongst other experiments they tried eliminating sleep altogether. The unsurprising result was that after only a few days the subjects became so disorientated that the experiments had to be stopped. Any moderately unscrupulous political interrogator throughout the centuries could have saved them the trouble, but it's nice to have these things scientifically certified.

More detailed experiments have shown that there are different levels of sleep and that it is most important to reach the deeper levels at least for short periods of time. In fact, even a healthy person does not reach the really deep levels for any great length of time, but if a person does not reach them at all, then slowly mental and emotional deterioration will take place. When people get to this stage, they turn to doctors for help and the medical profession prescribes literally mountains of pills. Many of these pills are entirely unnecessary; just a little common sense is all that is needed.

Your brain does not close down when you go to sleep. Far from it: this is the time when it does much of its most valuable work, but to do it, it needs peace and quiet. Internal peace and external quiet. Unlike your eyes, your ears cannot shut down. They remain open and fully operational while you are asleep. This is a part of your personal security system and therefore the messages that are sent in have a very high priority. Every time a message comes in you are prevented from going down into the important deep level of sleep, and a really urgent message can bring you up almost instantly from the deepest level.

For example, a woman can sleep quite well with trains running nearby all through the night, but a tiny whimper from her baby and she will be awake in an instant. This shows that it is the importance of the message which matters, rather than the quantity of messages. Now, the same thing applies to the internal messages. It is not the message, but the importance that you personally give to it. For example, no man is likely to be kept awake by the knowledge that he is going to have to mow the lawn in the morning, but the knowledge that if he cannot keep up his mortgage payments he will not have a lawn to mow will have a quite different priority rating.

The problem may be entirely different. Perhaps a matter of personal relationships. And the thing you are thinking about may have taken place years before. You are not aware of all these heart searchings, and the problem of raising them to your consciousness is dealt with in another chapter.

The way to go to sleep is firstly to make sure that as many of the physical conditions as possible are working in your favour, and then to create for yourself a going-to-sleep pattern.

Obviously from what has already been said, it is important to have as quiet a place to sleep as you can find. Now this is not always easy to come by in big cities because big cities seldom sleep. There is always something going on, from the road sweeper to the police siren and the noisy late-night drunk. If the level of noise is too high for you to deal with, then you have little option but to try and shut it out in some way. A clear conscience, of course, will change the sound of a police siren from an emergency signal to something you do not have to worry about, but it does seem that anything, if it is loud enough, will have some adverse effect.

Signals about your physical condition come from sources other than your ears. You can sense if you are getting too hot or too cold. During sleep the body sweats and consequently the bed coverings, the

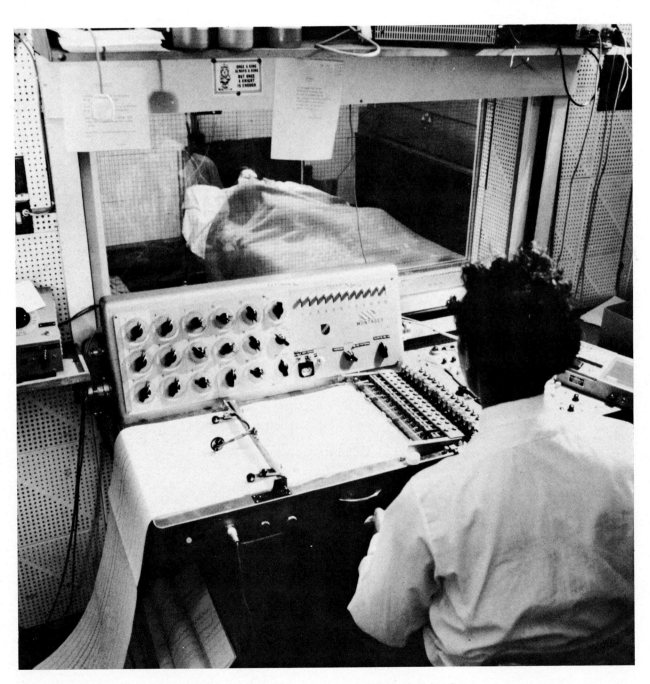

Sleep, it seems, is not quite the restful process it was once thought to be. At Edinburgh University
Sleep Research Centre, a doctor monitors the ECG machine which is recording the active brainwaves
of a sleeping subject who is outwardly peaceful.

sheets or blankets, should be porous and light and, if it is possible, you should sleep "in the raw", without nightclothes, so that the air can circulate around your body.

If you have central heating, this is no great problem, but in cold climates with less sophisticated home comforts it is less easy. However, there is one traditional system of keeping warm and at the same time having light bedclothes and no nightwear that has been handed down for centuries, especially in the eastern part of Europe where the cold winds sweep in from the Russian steppes. It is the traditional fairy-tale eiderdown. A big bag filled with the fine feathers of the eider duck and fitted with a slipover cover–this is all the bed covering you need. The true eiderdown can be fluffed up until it is maybe more than a foot thick. It fits round the body of the sleeper and gives a lightweight covering that allows you to sleep warm and cosy in the iciest of weather. The eiderdown cover is changed in the same way as ordinary bedsheets.

Cut down on one other source of disturbances, your stomach. Do not go to bed on a heavy meal. It may make you feel sleepy but it will not give you a good rest. Too much work will be going on in your body.

Eliminating any one condition is not likely to cure insomnia but if you put them all together they add up to a potentially effective sleep pattern. If you don't believe this, try putting the whole process into reverse. Ask yourself how much chance of a good night's sleep does somebody have if he is cold, has a bed in a room overlooking a noisy street, and has indigestion after a heavy meal at which he has been entertaining a business associate who, he hopes, is going to get him backing for a loan which will get him out of trouble at the bank. Any more for insomnia?

Now for the sleep pattern. Going to sleep is something that you can get to work on some time before you actually go to bed. The thing to do is to get your mind into the idea and the habit of sleep. Establish a routine which quite literally ends up with you going to sleep. As much as an hour before you want to go to sleep, shut yourself off from mental stimulation. This means turning off the television and not reading books late at night, especially those with which it is easy to identify. Make yourself ready for bed, always doing everything in the same order. Have a Hatha Yoga session if you are already into this way of life. Finish with a short meditation so that the mind is stilled and calmed, ready for your rest. Get into your night things, climb into bed, and turn out the light in the belief that every step is taking you nearer to sleep. Actually say this to yourself as you do it. It will take time for a pattern like this to be established, but when it is you will find yourself beginning to yawn before you are halfway through.

Once you are actually lying in bed, the technique is much the same as that used in total relaxation and is described fully on page 104. It is called 'yoga nidra', which means the yogic sleep. In true yoga nidra, you remain conscious while creating a total relaxation for yourself, but the same process can lead you to sleep.

All you have to do is become conscious of your body and then consciously relax it, starting from your toes and fingers and working gradually inwards and upwards to your face and your head. When you reach your head, you transfer your consciousness to

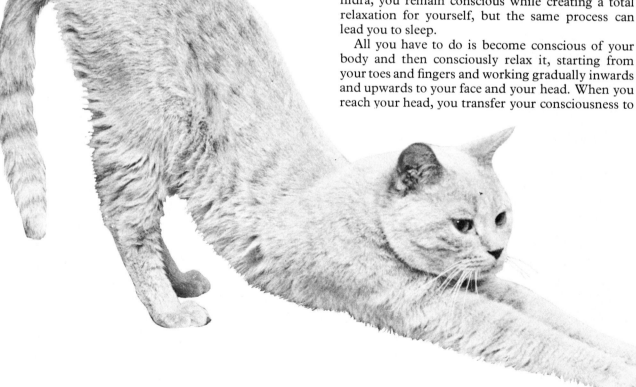

your breathing. Do not think about going to sleep; think only of the breath going quietly in and out through your nostrils. The more you concentrate on this and your total relaxation, the more easily you will go to sleep. The more your mind has been stilled before you go to sleep, the deeper you will sleep, and eventually the less sleep you will need. Ultimately you will be able to put yourself to sleep simply by thinking of your sleep routine. You'll say to yourself, 'Sleep time', while thinking of the routine you use – and that will be it.

Once in deep sleep, you should rise from it gradually, like a diver rising from a great depth. If an alarm clock pulls you out of deep sleep, it does act quite literally as an alarm. Your glands and nervous system are hurled into action and you use an enormous amount of your energy in coping with the violence of your awakening. If you really must use an alarm clock, then set it to go off ten minutes before you need to rise so that you can take your time in following your getting-out-of-bed routine.

You can learn the whole yogic system of waking up simply by watching a cat. Except in an emergency, a cat will never immediately leap into action on waking. None of this 'Hup! two, three. Who's for a cold bath?' First one eye will open and then the other and then there is a whole routine of stretching and yawning before that cat is good and ready for the first business of the day, which is usually a quick wash.

You should follow the same routine. If your alarm has woken you, turn it off without opening your eyes. Relax, because that alarm will have tensed you. Concentrate wholly on just lying there relaxed. Do not think yet about what is in the coming day. Open first one eye, then the other. Now a good general stretch. Lift your arms over your head, point your toes and – stretch. Have a deliberate yawn, bring your arms down, and lie quietly for a minute or two. The whole routine should be done slowly and should never take much less than three minutes.

Get out of bed but don't rush about. You are not finished yet. Stand by your bed and shake yourself. First, your arms; then your legs.

By this time it is quite possible that you feel the need for a bowel movement. Don't hold back on this, even though it means breaking into the rest of the routine. Inner cleanliness is very highly rated in Yoga. Next you must cleanse your mouth and brush your teeth. Yogis recommend scraping that white fur off the tongue with the edge of a spoon before the final rinse-out.

Early in the morning while your stomach is still empty is one of the best times of the day for a Hatha Yoga session. Half an hour of Yoga asanas will refresh you, whereas the hup-down-hup type of daily dozen is likely only to tire you, the reason being simply that Yoga asanas are designed primarily to promote health and not merely to build muscle. The daily dozen may be harder work, but this does not mean that you are doing yourself more good. Then, after half an hour (or more) of asanas, take a period of quiet meditation in which you clear your mind and review what the day will bring.

Now all this takes time, and you say you haven't got time. For one week try getting up half an hour earlier. Yoga asanas are boosters. They will more than make up for the half an hour in bed that you have lost. Of course, you could always go to bed half an hour earlier, and then you wouldn't lose anything at all.

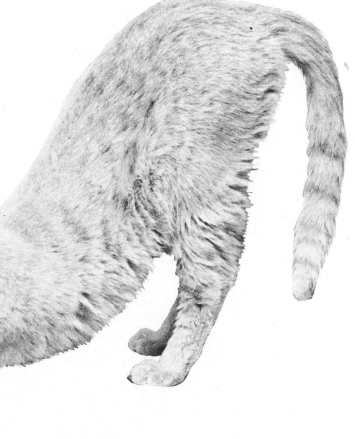

THE GOOD FOOD OF YOGA

you are what you eat – so eat well

If a yogi fasts it is for a limited period of time only and generally for the purpose of body cleansing; other than that, yogis insist on a good diet.

There are some yogis who appear almost literally to live on air, but this is simply because their stage of development and control enables them to use the prana in the food and air so efficiently that they live comfortably on a diet that would starve the average human. To give just two typical present-day examples: one, from India, is Hari Dass Baba, the teacher of Dr Richard Alpert, who eats so little that there are almost no wastes leaving his body; the other is an American yogini, Marcia Moore. As an impromptu experiment, Marcia Moore lived on an 800 calorie per day slimming diet. At the end of three weeks on a diet which would have knocked at least six to ten pounds off the average person, she had actually put *on* a pound and a half. Almost all yogis tend to eat rather less than average but they enjoy good food and a good appetite. At least two internationally famous yogis, Dr Mishra and B.K.S. Iyengar, are very good cooks who know well that the best food is food prepared with love.

The vast majority of yogis live on a lacto-vegetarian diet, that means a diet which is almost wholly fruit and vegetables but to which are added eggs and dairy products like butter or yoghurt. Very few of them are wholly vegans and very few of them eat meat, although there is no actual ban on meat eating.

Meat-eating yogis have a sound tradition on which to rely. Milarepa, the Tibetan yogi saint who lived at one time in an isolated mountain cave, was only too happy to abandon his temporary diet of nettle soup and eat meat, his body incidentally having turned green from his unadulterated diet of nettle broth.

'On partaking of the food, I enjoyed a sense of bodily ease and comfort, and a cheerfulness of mind that tended to increase my devotional exercises ... the meat I used sparingly until it was at last full of maggots ... Zezay again visited me bringing me a goodly supply of well cured meat and butter and a goodly supply of chang and flour ... I rejoiced at the prospect of having food such as ordinary human beings eat.'

Any modern nutritionist could point out that the high-protein/high-calorie food which his family had brought to him was particularly suited to the mountain cold in which he was living. The fact also remains that the lush fruit and vegetables beloved of wholly vegetarian yogis are simply not to be found in the rock-bound heights of the Himalayas.

The ethics of killing to eat is something which must be worked out by each individual. Some will be like the actor the late George Arliss, who, on walking along the line to find out why his train had stopped, was so horrified by the suffering of the cattle being taken to slaughter that he touched no meat from that moment on. The hunters who supplied Milarepa with meat were not oblivious to the problem either since they asked him to pray for the absolution of the animals which they had killed for food. There is little doubt that the further one goes into the awareness states of Yoga, the more one becomes aware of the quality of life in other living things. So that in looking, for example, at a piece of steak, one tends to get an image not only of the steak but of the living, walking beast of which it was once part, an effect which distinctly diminishes one's enthusiasm for meat. However, not all people are affected in this way and not all climates are mild enough to suit a wholly vegetarian diet, though there is mounting evidence that a vegetarian diet is an extremely healthy one. If the vegetables are properly washed there is virtually no danger of collecting disease from them, whereas the same thing certainly cannot be said for meat. Cold cooked meat is the renowned lurking place of salmonella bacteria, and under the present forced-rearing systems there is an ever-increasing risk from the antibiotics and hormones which are pumped into the beasts.

As with so many aspects of Yoga, Western researchers eventually arrived at answers which the yogis had had for centuries. The father of all Western nutrition systems was a certain Sir Robert McCarrison who, because of his position as the head of the medical services under the British Raj, was able to use the whole of the Indian continent as a gigantic nutritional research laboratory. It was he who finally established connections not only between disease and diet but between types of diseases and types of diets. He proved in the laboratories what the yogis had always said, 'You are what you eat.' The basic rules which McCarrison laid down for healthy eating tallied with those of the yogis.

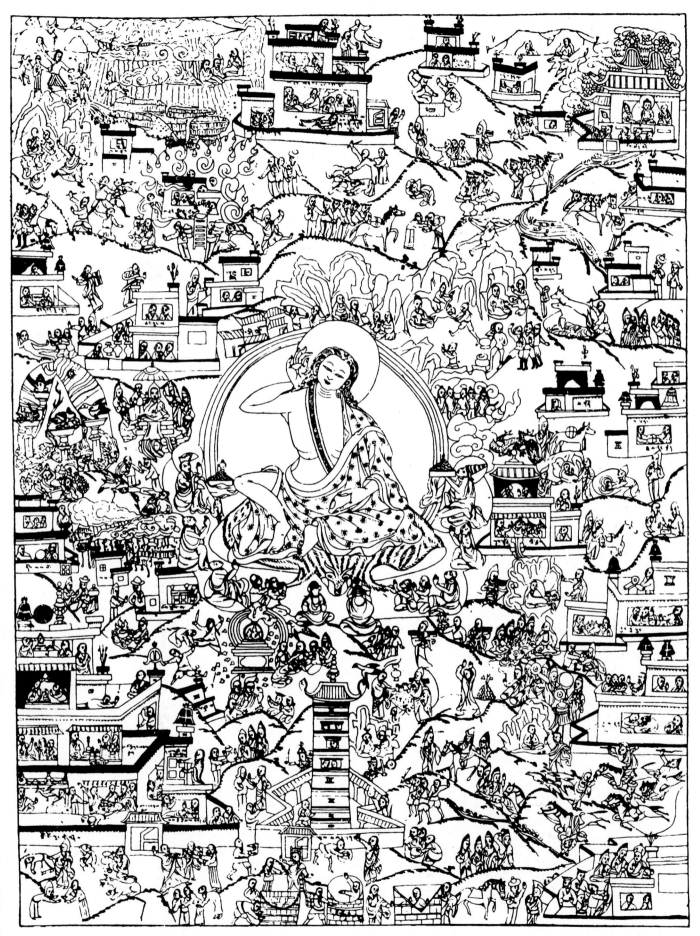

Milarepa, Tibet's most famous yogi, was a reformed eleventh-century black magician who founded one of Tibet's largest monasteries.

The rules are simple and in no way cranky. Basically you should eat moderately of a good well-mixed diet containing plenty of fresh organically grown fruit and vegetables. 'Organic' is taken to mean that they are grown under natural conditions in rich composted soil without the use of chemicals. Essentially yogic eating is a matter of quality before quantity. The most important divergence from routine Western diet is that all grains should be eaten whole. That is to say that rice, flour, and bread should not be white. They should always be whole-grain or brown. The modern high-speed flour mill was probably the biggest single nutritional disaster ever to strike the Western world. The grains are milled so finely that the 'germ' of the wheat, containing almost all the vitamins and food value, is removed from the flour. The biggest losses are in the Vit E and the Vit B complex.

Fortunately this disaster has been recognized and it is now possible in many places to buy brown flour, brown rice, barley, etc. through health stores. On the other hand, many supermarkets may not offer a single thing which is up to yogic standards, the shelves being filled with food which may once have been valuable but which has been so treated that almost all of its value has been lost to increase its 'shelf life'. In fact, the lunatic situation has arrived in which it is possible for a Western man to stuff himself so full of food that he has a continual weight problem, while at the same time suffering from chronic malnutrition owing to the lack of food value in the artificially treated bulk that he has been eating.

This situation is much more common than you might think – and the food manufacturers are not the only miscreants in the matter. What happens in a poorly conducted family kitchen will remove any last remaining scrap of life force in the food. Good cooking can increase the ease with which the body can absorb certain vital substances from the food. Bad cooking destroys these substances. The safest rule about cooking is – don't. It is amazing what can be eaten raw, once you get used to the idea and learn to appreciate the existence of a whole new set of tastes.

Yogis divide food into three categories:

1. sattvic
Sattvic food is considered the ideal food for the yogi. It should be mild, fresh and nutritious. A sattvic food is one which would be found in a lacto-vegetarian diet but with the following difference. The sattvic vegetables and fruits are generally those which are grown above the surface of the ground, where they are subject to the vitalizing rays of the sun. Such foods include peas, beans, lettuce, cabbage, apples, figs, nuts, and whole grains. Yoghurts and honey are also sattvic foods.

2. rajasic
Rajasic foods are those which the yogis consider will make you more earthy or passionate and include red meats and root crops, such as carrots, potatoes, and so on. Into this rajasic group also come spices, salts, peppers and anything which has a very strong taste. Fish and chicken can be either sattvic or

rajasic, apparently according to how a person feels about flesh eating.

3. tamasic
It is only in this area that the yogis and the Western dieticians differ. Most Westerners believe in the use of offal, the livers and kidneys of beasts. Yogis dismiss these items as being unhealthy to eat. In hot climates, this is probably a wise rule, but it is possibly less necessary in cooler regions. However, there is no doubt that while liver and kidneys contain certain vitamins in concentration, they are also very prone to contain bacteria. On the whole, it would seem that if you are prepared to eat meat at all, you might as well go all the way and eat the offal as well.

Two other items on the tamasic list which may cause consternation in the Western cook are onions and garlic. However, Western gourmets will be glad to know that these are not universally disapproved. In fact at least one sect of Yoga teachers is firmly in favour of garlic. It is after all a natural disinfectant and a blood purifier, even if it may be unwelcome on the astral plane – it is in relation to transcendental awareness that garlic is thought to be undesirable.

There is a difference between eating and just stoking up. Yogically speaking, eating and universal love are, or should be, inextricably combined. There is an old Sufi adage that food eaten with anger turns to poison. Food eaten without concentration is empty. Food eaten at a business lunch by politicians who smile while plotting each other's downfall can only breed ulcers and coronaries. If the man who grows the food loves it, that love goes with it; if the cook also loves it, so much the better. If you sit at a table and you are asked to pass someone a dish, then pass it with love. It costs you nothing and it's the finest investment you can make. If you cast your bread upon the waters, it frequently comes back buttered.

The label on the tin in the supermarket may be very pretty, and the supermarket itself the latest in hygiene and accounting efficiency – but what about the food? The over-centralization of cities has created probably the most inefficient nutritional system in the history of man. The more preservatives are added to a food and the longer the food takes to reach the consumer, the more its nutritional value decreases. Losses sometimes reach 90%. The most efficient nutritional system would probably be to have a kitchen garden attached to each family house so that the food could travel from the soil to the table in a matter of minutes.

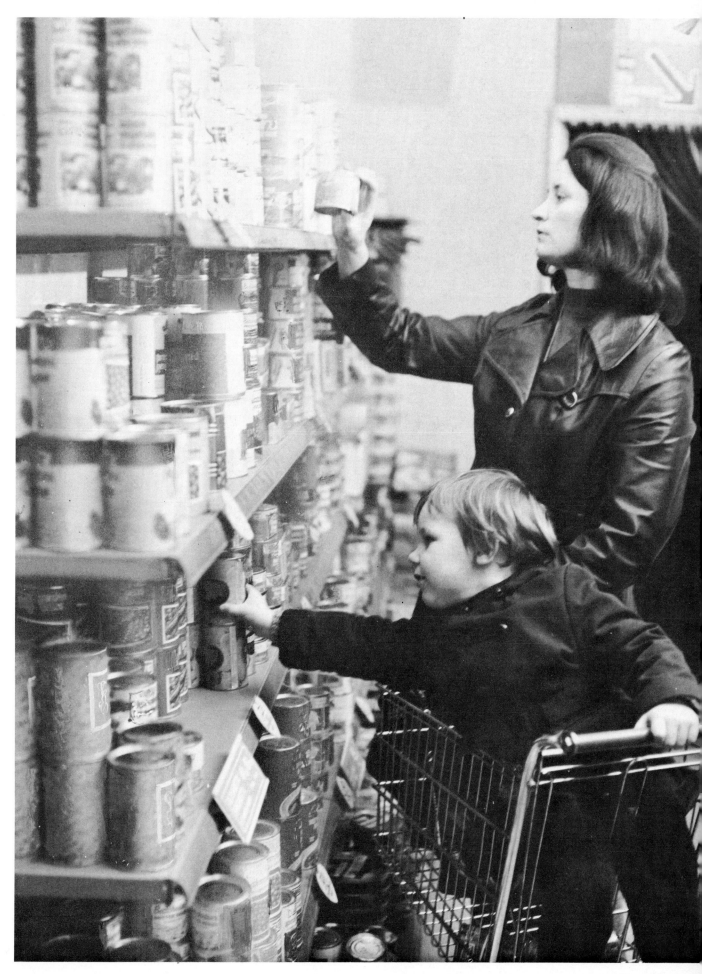

PRANAYAMA, THE BREATH OF LIFE

You are a living, pulsing, vibrating being. Stop breathing and you stop living. Learn to observe your breath and you learn to observe yourself and your moods. Control your breath and you control your moods. Try it. Instead of sitting quietly reading, put this book aside and begin to breathe jerkily and irregularly. Before long you will begin to feel edgy, uneasy, or even angry. Reverse the process and breathe slowly and quietly and evenly, and soon a sensation of peace will slide over you.

Good breathing is the first thing taught by any yogi, and nothing will give you so good a return for so little effort. Do not underestimate the power concealed in breathing. There are many unusual breathing patterns in Yoga, each with its own purpose, and so effective is controlled breathing that the techniques are considered by some to be best kept secret because of their strength.

Everyday breathing is usually left to haphazard control by the body's autonomic reflex and the unconscious mind. Pranayama, on the other hand, aims to bring the whole breathing system under conscious control. This is done by becoming intensely aware of the body mechanisms which are involved and by deliberately modifying the rhythms and force of the breathing.

For example, the lungs are consciously operated in the lower, middle, or upper lobes during exercises. By advanced techniques this can even be carried to the extent of operating a single lobe in either the right or the left lung. Rhythms are studied by dividing the action of breathing into these categories:

Puraka . . . inhalation
Kumbhaka . . . held-in-breath
Rechaka . . . exhalation
Shunyaka . . . held-out breath

Obviously an enormous variety of breathing patterns can be achieved. Swami Yogeswarananda considers that there are fifty classical pranayama, let alone the many variations devised from time to time by individual yogis. For beginners, the patterns are based on a count of three, to match the three lobes of the lungs. A typical first exercise would be 3 in–6 out, the exhalation being twice as long as the inhalation. The count could be increased very gradually until it became 10 in–20 out, when it would be classified as a 'butterfly breath' (a pattern in which the ingoing and outgoing breath of the yogi is so slow that it creates no more sound or disturbance than the wings of a butterfly).

Holding the breath either in or out is considered to be tremendously important, but the technique is introduced only after regular in and out breathing is thoroughly under control. Then, a simple pattern of 3 in–3 hold–3 out–3 hold could be used, 3–3–3–3. One classical pattern is 1–4–2–4, but this is recommended only under supervision because any increase in the first figure, the inhalation, brings such an enormous increase in the holding figures. All patterns should be extended only very slowly over many months.

Breaths used to cleanse the body or the nerve channels tend to reverse the 3–6 pattern to something like 3–1, the breath being drawn in very slowly and then exhaled very sharply often with a 'Ha' sound. In this technique the arms are often raised above the head as the breath is taken in, then sharply brought down so that they help to force the breath out completely with a 'Ha!'.

Most yogic breathing is carried out using a complete breath. This is not quite the same as a deep breath. A complete breath involves all of the stale air being forced out of the lungs before the fresh air is drawn in, and the whole of the torso being free to participate in the breath.

The majority of people in the West suffer from a form of "frozen torso", in which they try to breathe without moving either their ribs or their stomach properly. This is largely due to our inhibited outlook on sex. Breathing is a natural rhythmic action which should involve the entire torso. Unfortunately, most of us in the West have been brought up to think of sex as sinful and to believe that any awareness in the area of the sex organs, and this includes the lower part of the abdomen, is "naughty, naughty". The result is very simply that any breathing which tends to include a movement in the lower part of the torso has been damped down and the breathing action has been confined to the upper part of the ribs, which, being a "clean", "pure" area and as far away from the sex organs as possible, is permitted to move without guilt. In the case of some people, this reaction is so ingrained that it is first necessary to establish the idea not merely that the abdomen should move–but that it *can* move.

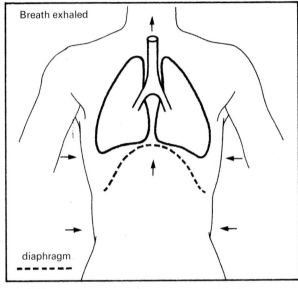

Breath inhaled

Note the diaphragm movement

Breath exhaled

diaphragm

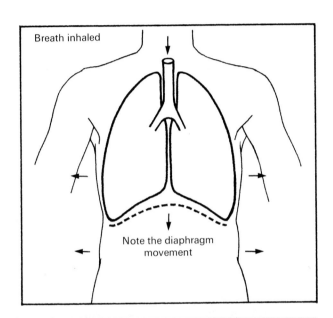

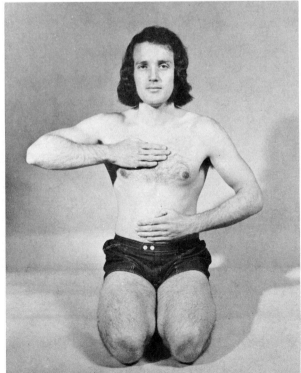

Place the hands on the chest and on the abdomen in order to check for a correct breathing movement.

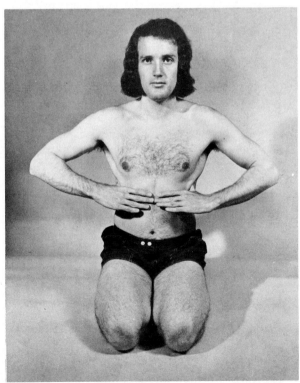

To encourage expansion of the lower ribs, place the hands so that the fingers touch when the breath is squeezed out. The hands should part as you breathe in.

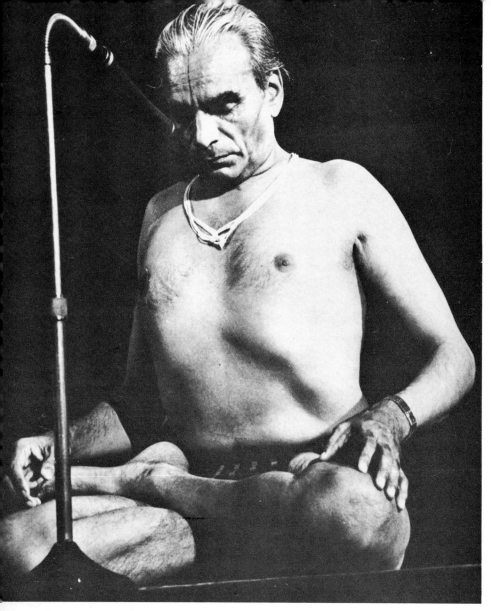

Left: B.K.S. Iyengar uses a microphone to demonstrate the characteristic hissing sound made by Ujjayi, a long slow breath. This sound is almost the hallmark of a well-trained yogi because, although Ujjayi is not difficult to do, it is almost impossible to learn it without the supervision of a good teacher. The air is drawn in very slowly while the back of the throat is slightly contracted; this makes the characteristic hissing sound. When the lungs are well filled, the breath is held for a short period and then slowly released with the same sound, caused by the constriction of the soft palate. There is a very short pause and the breath is drawn in again, and so on. An ideal tranquillizer and cleanser, this pranayama can be practised at any time of the day or night. Below: Some beginners cannot relax their torsos while sitting up so for them breathing is begun lying down. Opposite: The Complete Breath Standing.

The simplest breathing exercise is called the **Complete Breath Lying Down.** Lie on the floor on your back with your knees bent, place your hands on your ribs and check if you can feel them moving when you breathe. Next place your hands in the arch of the ribs and breathe very deeply in and out. As you breathe out, so you squeeze the air out with your hands. Continue breathing until you can feel the whole of your body contracting and expanding as the air goes in and out. Then take your hands away and breathe to your own natural rhythm. This means that you observe your own breathing reflex and breathe only when it demands. Breathe out and make no attempt to breathe in until your body demands it. Then breathe in really deeply. Breathe out again only when your body tells you to. You will find that your body pauses for longer when your lungs are empty than when they are full. At this point make no attempt to force your breathing into any specific pattern. Concentrate on making sure that *all* of the air goes out of your lungs, and they will refill entirely automatically.

This is natural breathing and it is the pattern of breathing you should use when you are holding any completed Yoga posture unless instructed other-

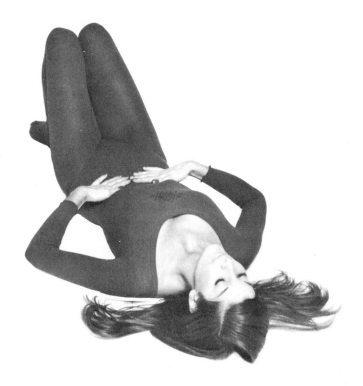

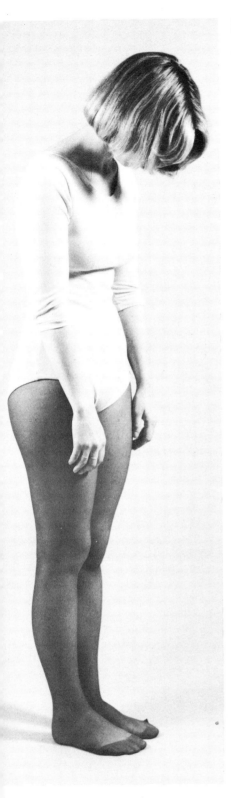
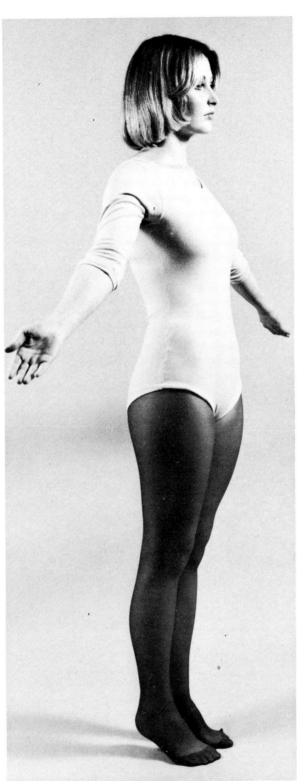
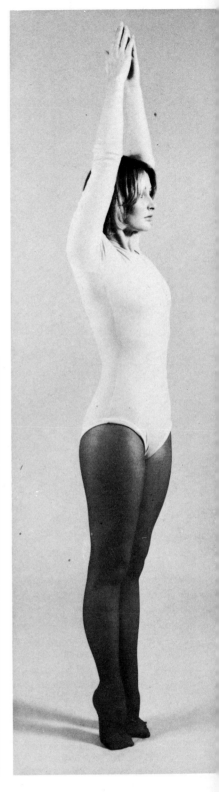

wise. The basic rule for linking breathing to postures is that as you bend, you breathe out, when you hold the posture you breathe naturally, and as you straighten up the torso, you breathe in. Certain forms of Yoga demand more precisely controlled patterns of breathing but this basic rule will hold good for virtually all asanas.

The **Complete Breath Standing** is an example of simple forced breath in Yoga. Stand with your head dropped forward and your hands hanging by your sides. Breathe out. Then slowly raise your arms, palms up. At the same time raise yourself on tiptoe and breathe slowly in so that your lungs are full when your hands meet above your head. Pause on tiptoe and turn your hands palms outwards. Now slowly lower your arms, sink back on your heels and let the last of your breath out as you reach your starting position. Repeat this slowly several times, trying very hard to synchronize all your movements.

This exercise helps you to breathe using the ribs.

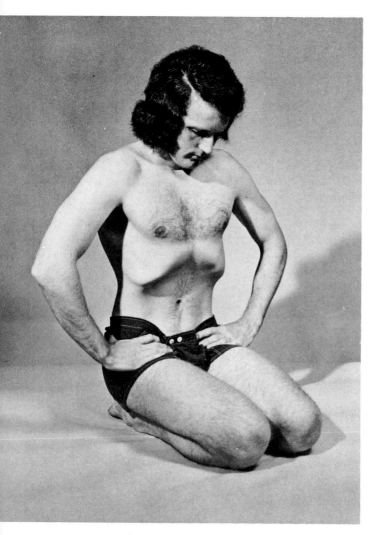

Uddiyana is strictly speaking a 'bandha', or lock, but it is often used in pranayamas and is excellent for creating an awareness of the diaphragm. First you exhale and hold the breath out. Then you expand the chest as though to draw in breath, but without taking in any air. This automatically sucks the stomach in and you then pull it back against the spine with the stomach muscles. Still holding the breath out, you can 'flap' the stomach in and out three or four times. Hold and then relax. This bandha is extremely effective for massaging the intestines.

Think of them expanding at the *sides and back* and learn to get this side/back expansion when you are breathing sitting down. Exercise breathing can be exaggerated, but normal breathing should only be deep. Always concentrate on getting the stale air out.

When you feel that your torso is beginning to unfreeze and your breathing is becoming deeper, you can sit cross-legged or in Vajrasana (see page 64) and practise breathing with any one part of your ribs or torso. For example, to check on rib breathing put your hands on the lower-back ribs and concentrate on making them move in and out. Alternatively, place your hand on the upper front ribs and try to get the maximum movement out of that area for a while. After any forced breathing always have a period in the relaxed natural rhythm to stabilize yourself.

A typical forced breath which will require you to stabilize if it is overused is **Bhastrika**, the **Bellows Breath**. This is an excellent breath for generally cleansing the system and it consists in pumping the breath in and out very vigorously and rapidly, visualizing dirty air going out and clean air and prana coming in. Start with a few rounds of Bhastrika and build up the number very slowly. It is very easy to become oxy-drunk from the additional

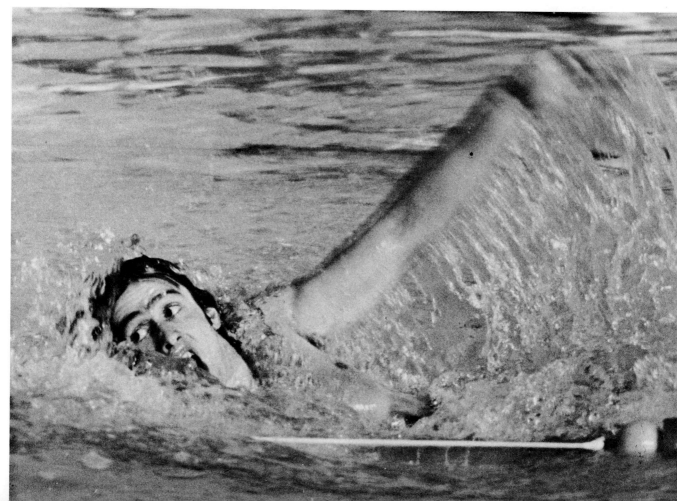

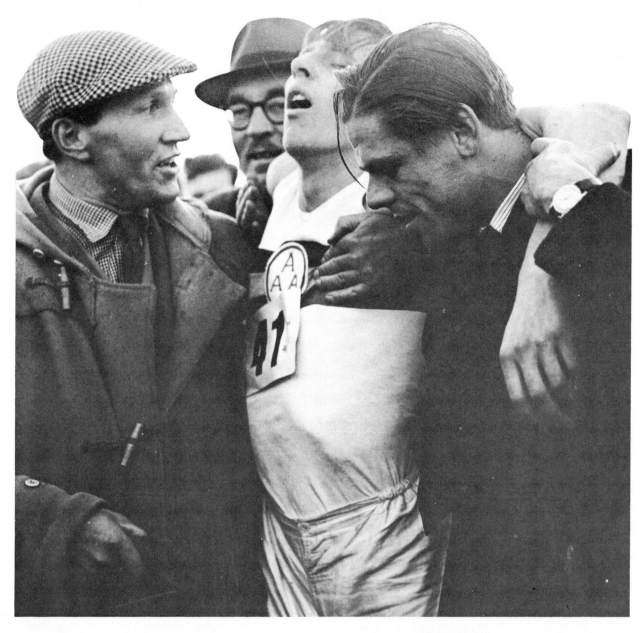

Opposite: Swimming is probably the only sport in which the breath is brought under a very rhythmic control as in Yoga.

Above: Typical athlete's exhaustion. Dr Roger Bannister, world record miler, had to make good an enormous oxygen loss.

amount of oxygen that is taken in, but the effect wears off very quickly.

This breath illustrates the value of Yoga Pranayama. Most panting breaths are necessity breaths. You pant after exercise because your body is in desperate need of oxygen. In sport all you are doing is making good a loss, whereas in yogic panting, which is done quite voluntarily and without necessity, you are recharging yourself to a high level. This is simply because you are not starting off from a point of exhaustion as an athlete does.

With all the Yoga pranayamas, the effect can be modified according to the mental direction of the prana. You visualize force coming into you as you breathe in, and as you breathe out you visualize that force flowing from your solar plexus to the area of your body where you wish to direct it. Such a visualization has a recharging effect. Breathing can also be used to "magnetize" the body prior to really advanced techniques. However, neither of these

techniques can be approached until a firm control has been established over your breathing.

Pranayama, the direction of life force by breathing, is powerful stuff. It should be taken in small doses but regularly. It is the regularity which enables you to make changes in yourself. The rule about whether you have had enough is simple: if you have to think about it then you have had enough.

why yogis sit cross legged

Why do yogis sit cross legged? The answer is simply that the yogic system was created thousands of years ago, mostly in a country where people were used to sitting on cushions on the floor. If you really do not want to sit cross legged to do meditation, then you can do it perfectly well in a chair. In fact, if you are really stiff you will be better off in a chair.

However, since many of the exercises were devised for someone sitting in the cross-legged position, it is much easier to follow them if you develop the habit of sitting this way. There is another – and practical – reason for sitting cross legged. All of the traditional writings on Yoga stress the importance of sitting with the spine in as erect a position as possible. Patanjali said:

'Sitting is to be steady and pleasurable. This is done by loosening of effort and by thinking on the endless (infinity).'

From the purely yogic point of view there is yet another and important reason to sit cross legged. Prana flows round the body and tends to escape at the fingers and the feet. If the hands and legs are crossed or folded, especially as in the Lotus Seat, then a "closed circuit" of energy is formed, minimizing the leak of life energy by continually feeding it back into the body.

If you can master the Lotus Seat *easily*, then it can be remarkably comfortable. But there are many who, because of their build and because they did none of these things in childhood, will never be able to do the Lotus in comfort. It is of no importance. Many of the other easier sitting positions have closely similar effects.

In fact, even in India a great many adepts prefer to use a posture known as Siddhasana. So far as the traditional yogis are concerned, the only real advantage of the Lotus Seat is that it is a 'locked' posture, which means that the legs cannot slip apart, and hence one cannot overbalance if in a deep trance. Modern yogis, such as Dr Mishra, place less importance on this and say that it is enough to be adequately propped up on a chair so long as the spine is held straight.

The instructions from the *Hatha Yoga Pradipika* on how to do **Padmasana** or the **Lotus Seat** are beautifully simple.

'Place the right foot on the left thigh, and the left foot on the right thigh. Place the chin on the chest and gaze at the tip of the nose...'

It's that simple – but not that easy!

The trouble of course lies in getting the foot onto the thigh and, even if you can do that, sliding the second foot over the opposite knee appears at first sight to be a total impossibility to the majority of people. The obvious difficulty is in getting the knees flat enough and this can only be tackled by working at increased suppleness from the waist downward. This point must be understood because the consulting rooms of osteopaths have been filling with a new malady which is first cousin to tennis elbow. It is being christened "yoga knee" and is the result of people trying to force themselves into the Lotus Posture before they are ready for it. If the

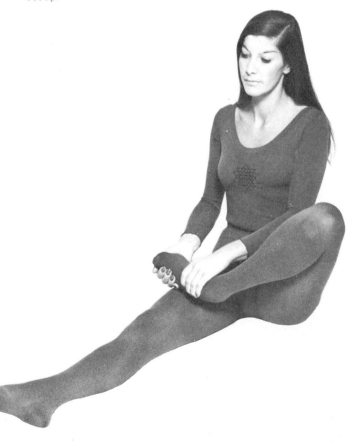

Padmasana, the Lotus Seat. Never, never force this posture: damaged knees often do not recover. Turn the sole of the foot up.

hips and ankles are not supple enough, then almost all the leverage is concentrated on the knee joint with the inevitable result that it gets damaged. Once it is damaged, it can take a very long time to recover and can prevent the comfortable use of folded-leg postures permanently.

Many stretching exercises which would appear to have little to do with cross-legged postures do in fact affect your ability to do them. For example Mr Iyengar's Standing Stretches (Trikonasana etc.) are extremely useful for exercising those areas which need to be stretched for the Lotus and similar postures (see page 60).

Another exercise which is a good preparation for cross-legged sitting is the Alternate Leg Stretch on page 69.

An exercise directly related to the Lotus Seat is called **Bhadrasana** or the **Knee and Thigh Stretch** (see page 61). It is very simple to perform and so easy to control that the amount of stretch which you apply need never cause a strain. Sit with your legs straight out in front of you. Lean forward and, cupping your hands over your feet, press the soles together and slowly draw the feet as close in to your body as you can manage. At the same time allow the knees to fall outward as far as possible. The eventual aim is that you should be easily able to touch the pelvic bone with your heels, and your legs should lie completely flat along the floor with the knees touching the ground. Some people are unusually flexible and will be able to do this immediately, but the vast majority of adults will need many months, even years, before their legs drop completely horizontal. Some teachers advocate bobbing the knees up and down to increase the stretching effect, but be careful as it is only too easy

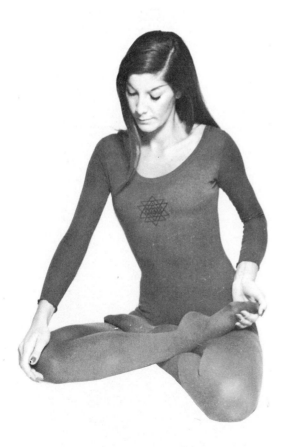

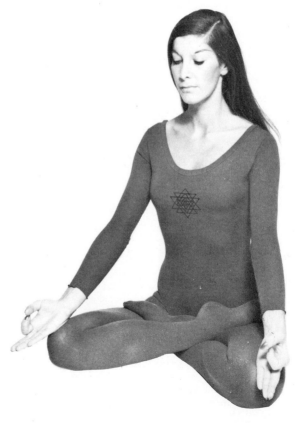

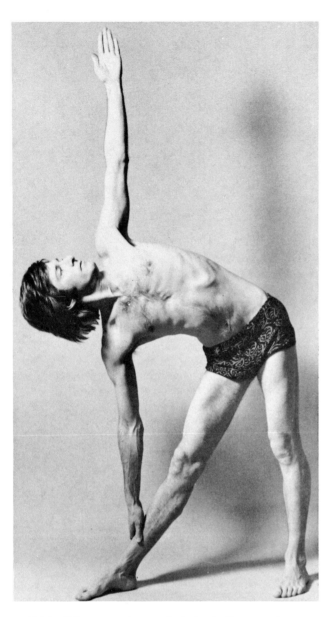

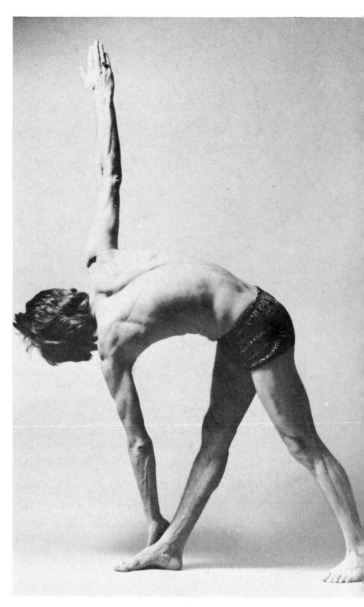

Utthitta Trikonasana, the stretched triangle. Have your feet apart, your arms raised to shoulder level. When bending to the right, turn the right foot 90 degrees to the right, the left foot only slightly. Exhale and bend sideways, if possible touching the floor with your fingers. Try to extend the body as you bend; do not just crumple over. Hold for 30 seconds, breathing evenly, and come up on an inhalation. Repeat to the other side.

to acquire very sore ligaments on the inside of the legs which can retard your progress.

Rotation is another useful stretch, but it is not so very well known. Sit with both legs straight out in front of you. Bend one leg at the knee and hold it at the knee and the ankle. Rotate it as shown in the illustration. This is a very powerful stretch and must be used with discretion. The leg and the ankle must be relaxed and you can test this by shaking the leg. If you are tense, you will not be able to shake your foot.

If these last three movements are practised, together with your daily Yoga routine, then quite unexpectedly one day you will find that you can slide your foot up into your thigh for a short time in preparation for a Lotus. Do not be put off if nothing seems to happen for a long, long time. The

body does not improve an equal amount each day. On some days it merely stores the knowledge of its development and only when it has decided that it is safe to relax itself further will it "let go" and give you the extra movement. The improvement may be so slow that you can hardly see it on a daily or, possibly, weekly basis, but be assured that the less you try to force it, the quicker you will progress. Suppleness slowly achieved is likely to be permanent, whereas forced suppleness will not be. The body's memory will always classify it as "risky", whereas slow development will be "safe".

Opposite top: Utthitta Parsvakonasana, the stretched flank. Turn the feet as for Trikonasana, exhale, and bend the knee until it forms a right angle. Place one hand on the floor and bring the other arm over the head. Breathe deeply and stretch the whole of the body. Straighten up on an inhalation. Repeat to the other side.
Opposite, near right: Rotation. The aim of the exercise is to stretch the hip joint and pelvis, not the knee. Relax all the muscles, and, keeping the shin at the same angle all the time, rotate the whole of the lower leg. Never twist the knee; all the movement should be in the hip.

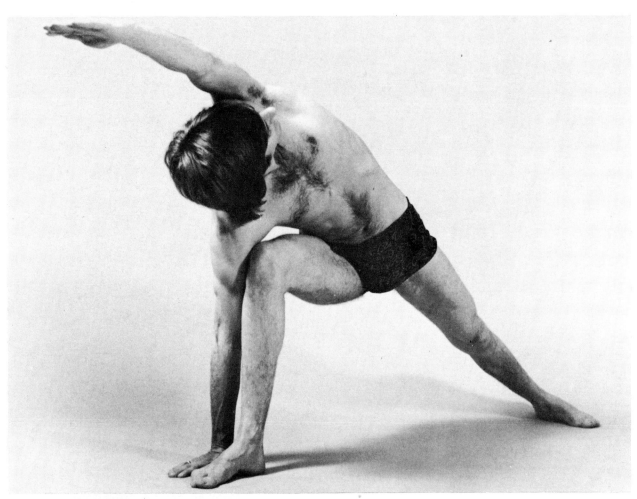

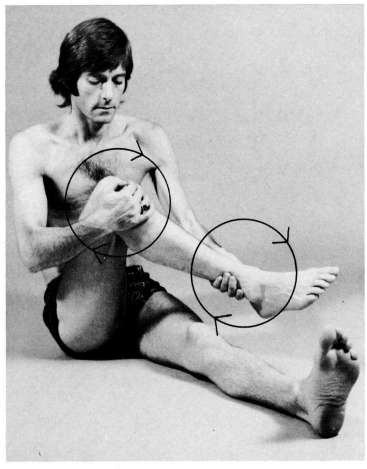

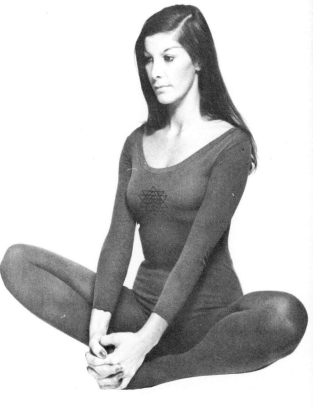

Bhadrasana, the Knee and Thigh Stretch. Move the knees gently up and down like butterfly wings.

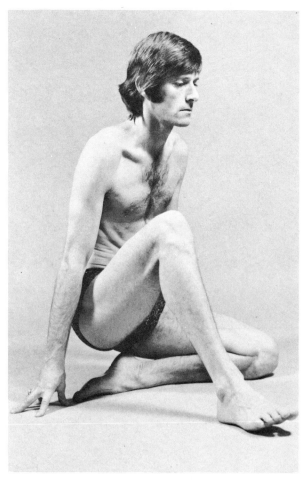

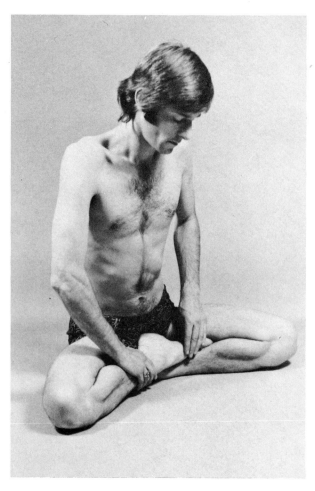

Siddhasana is favoured more by adepts than the Lotus Seat.

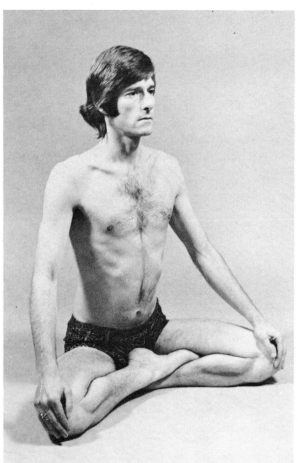

However, for some people it is better, for reasons of age or whatever, to accept that it is simply not worth the trouble for them to slave daily to get into the Lotus. Now this is no reason to feel that you are not being a yogi, that you are breaking thousands of years of tradition, or that you are a dismal failure and congenitally malformed. The inability of some people to do the Lotus has been recognized for thousands of years, and the little statuette illustrated here shows the ancient classic solution. The pose is called **Baddha Sukhasana**, the **Easy Bound**, or **Yoga Belt Pose**.

You must be comfortable to meditate. When the knees in any cross-legged pose are not supported by the ground, they become a focus of discomfort and intrude mercilessly on concentration. So to achieve relaxation, a wide band of cloth or a belt is fastened in a loop which passes completely round the body and supports the knees, thus allowing the user to relax completely against the loop while holding the spine more or less straight. Adjust the size of the loop to suit your own comfort and then simply slip it over your head and into position whenever you need it. Be sure that the loop is broad enough to be comfortable and not like a piece of rope, which, because it is narrow, will affect the circulation.

The use of the Yoga Belt is traditional where sitting on the ground is a domestic routine, but Dr Mishra has devised a chair pose which is equally

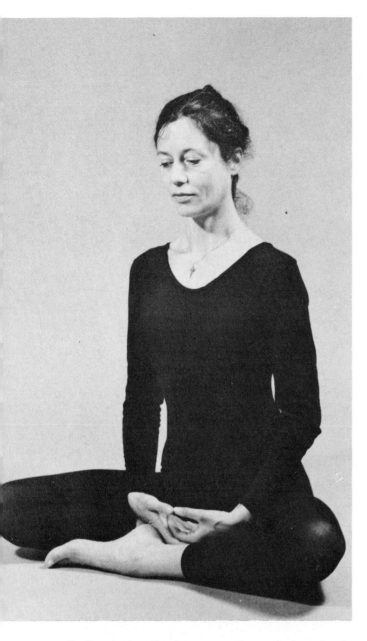

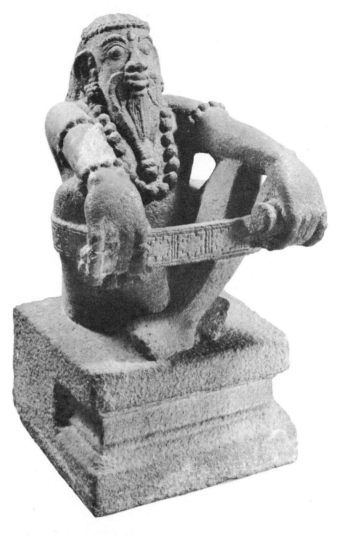

Any discomfort, even in Sukhasana *(left)*, makes meditation impossible. Hence the use of a band to take the strain, as in this small seventeenth-century stone statue *(above)* from Southern India.

effective as a meditative posture because the spine is held straight and one cannot fall over. It is also much easier for a Westerner, who is accustomed to sitting in chairs. This very familiarity with the chair helps to relax the mind.

The **Chair Pose** is more or less self explanatory. You sit in a well-padded armchair with your feet up on a stool in front of you. The legs are roughly at right angles to the body so that the spine is kept straight. The legs and hands can be crossed or not. The stool supporting the legs should be fairly close to the chair so that there is no strain on the knees. The position should be so comfortable that once you have settled into it, there is no need to move for a very considerable time.

For anyone who feels that a chair pose is too much of a break with tradition, there are three other seated Yoga postures. They are: Siddhasana, Sukhasana, and Vajrasana.

Begin **Siddhasana, the Pose of an Adept,** by sitting on the floor with your legs straight out in front of you. Draw in one foot until the heel is just under

the centre of the pubic bone. Now draw in the other foot, turning the sole up so that the foot rests in the fold of the other leg. Both heels should be on the centre line of the body. Practise this alternately, having the left foot underneath and then changing and having the right one underneath. It needs a certain amount of practice but it is much easier than the Lotus.

Sukhasana, the **Easy Pose,** can be achieved by almost anyone, though it will not necessarily be comfortable at first. Sit with your legs crossed. Take hold of your feet and draw them as far under you as they will comfortably go. Let your knees relax so that they fall outwards and sit as upright as possible. Both of these poses can be made easier by sitting on a cushion or a couple of books. As your suppleness increases, so you will be able to use a thinner book or less cushion. You can gradually sit nearer and nearer to the front edge of the cushion until you can dispense with it entirely if you wish. But there is no reason why you shouldn't have some sort of a cushion for meditating.

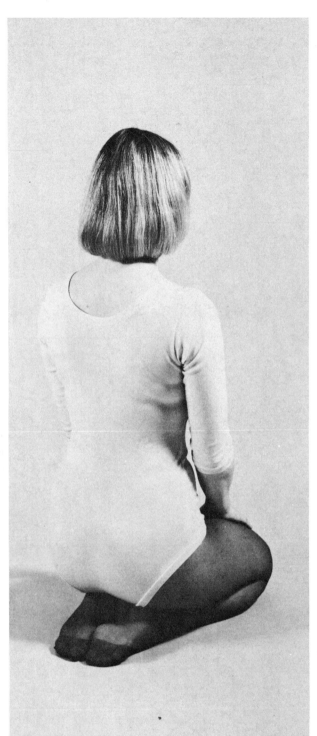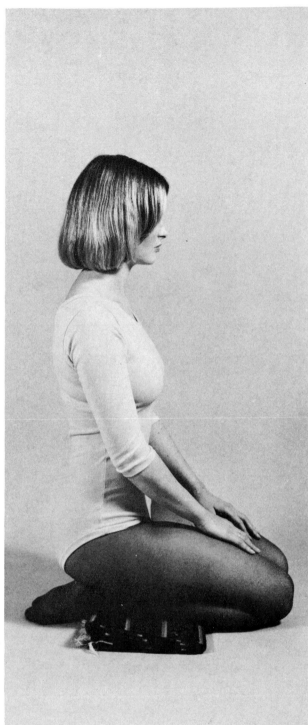

Vajrasana, the Thunderbolt Pose, is probably the most neglected posture in Yoga.

Finally there is **Vajrasana,** the **Thunderbolt** or **Pelvic Pose,** in which you kneel down and then sit back on your heels, a form of sitting which is very commonly used domestically in Japan. Apart from being very suitable for meditation, this posture is reputed to have an excellent effect on the digestion. As the ancient yogis put it, 'It increases the digestive fires.' For some reason, women seem to be able to adopt this posture very much more easily than most men. It needs suppleness in the knees and ankles, but relatively little in the hips. If you are not able to assume this position easily, then do not risk straining your knees. Place a small cushion beneath your shins or in between your legs and sit on that until you have become used to the posture.

Vajrasana is an extremely useful and comfortable posture and yogically speaking it is very efficient. It provides a satisfactory answer for many people who would otherwise find themselves depressingly uncomfortable in the folded-leg postures and who would lose valuable time trying to make themselves comfortable. Most exercises performed in the Lotus Seat could just as appropriately be performed in Vajrasana.

THE ASANAS

Yoga's effortless exercises

In the yogic way of life, there are very few yogis who do not practice the asanas. The word 'asana' means seat or posture and it is this static quality that makes the exercises so different from the Western jump-and-bend type of gymnastics.

It matters not whether you are bound on a spiritual path or purely on improving yourself physically, the asanas serve a purpose. So, as a yogi, your day is likely to begin with anything from ten to thirty minutes (or even more) of asanas. As you progress you may find that you can maintain your physical standards with a shorter and shorter period. It is quite customary for the dignified heads of ashrams in India to come out on their verandahs and spend a quiet twenty minutes performing their "daily dozen". But in their case they will have developed such experience and concentration that they will be able to get as much out of their twenty minutes as most people would get out of an hour of practice.

In contrast to these few minutes spent daily by the teachers, some chelas may spend almost their whole day on asanas and vigorous exercises. The late Professor Barnard, when he went to study in the Himalayas, found himself doing three and four hours a day and repeating particular exercises hundreds of times until the perspiration flowed off him. Right away let it be clear that this sort of intense training is not to be undertaken except with the proper supervision. There is no quicker way of upsetting your system than to plunge sweatily headfirst into hours of exhausting practice. An experienced teacher can see the signs of strain and unbalance appearing in the student long before the student becomes aware of them and will reduce his work accordingly.

If you have the slightest doubt about your work load, then reduce it. The reason for this care is that almost all of the asanas tend to build energy rather than expend it. This of course explains the lift that Yoga will give you, in contrast to jump-and-bend sports, which leave you exhausted. With Yoga exercises pumping extra energy into you, you have to allow time for your whole organism to adapt itself to taking the extra load before you can put that energy to full use. In the beginning you should hold the various positions for what may seem a quite uselessly short time, only a few seconds. Increase the amount of time very gradually and very regularly.

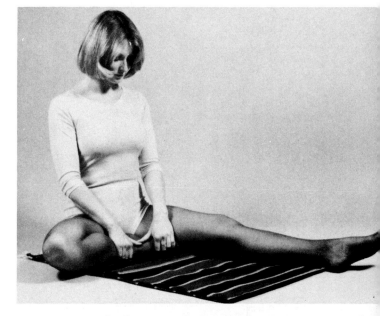

Beginning Janu Sirsasana, the Alternate Leg Stretch.

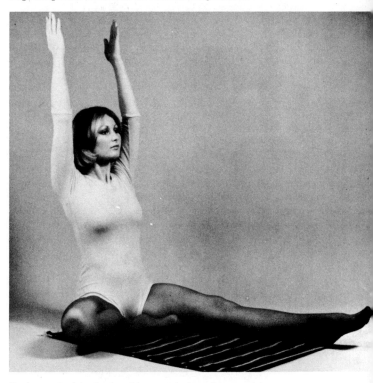

Having tucked the heel well in, stretch the spine upwards.

65

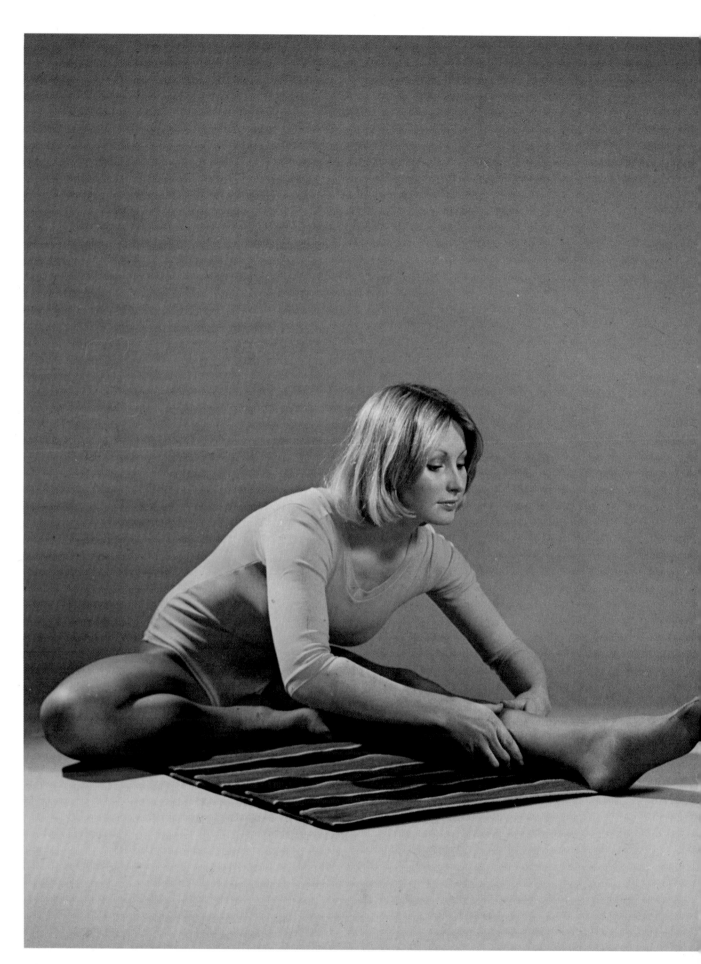

At first you may only be able to progress this far.

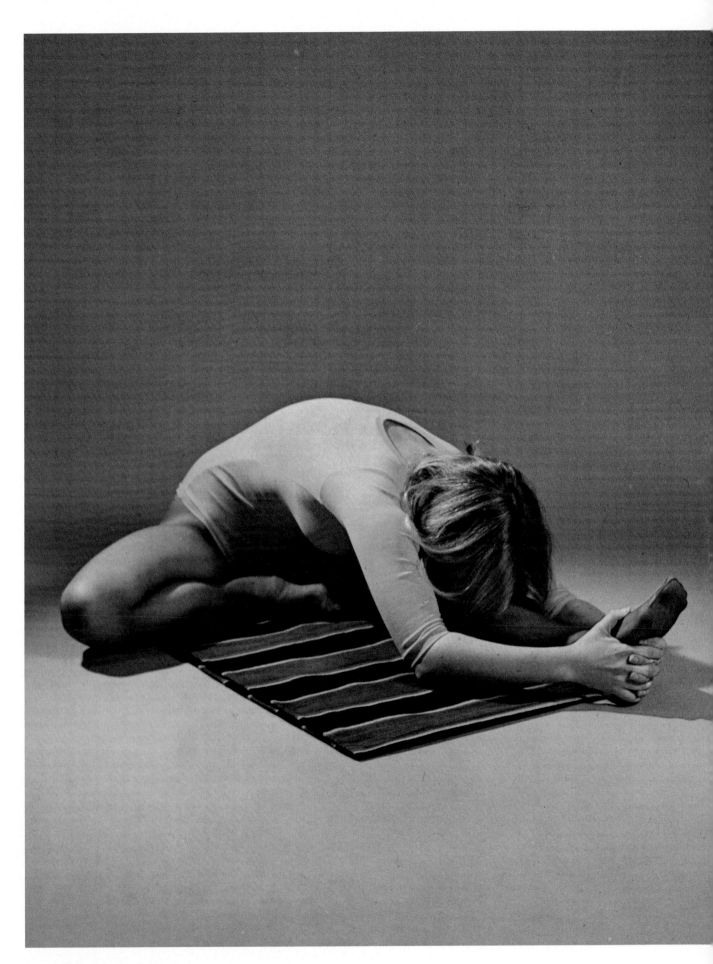

As you gradually become expert, so you bend further forward.

Below: Janu Sirsasana, an alternative method for beginners.

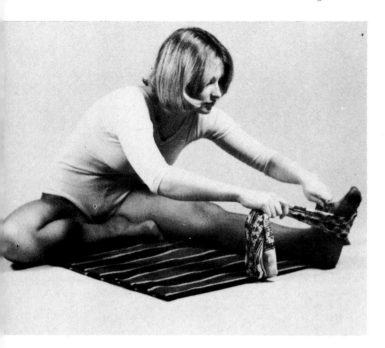

Below: Starting the Paschimottanasana, the Back Stretch.

Once you have gone through your getting-up routine you are ready for your morning asana session. Be sure that your body is warm and that you have a rug to lie on and plenty of fresh air. Some people like to use a very thin sheet of foam plastic. Whatever you use, it should be thick enough only to take the discomfort out of the hard floor. If it is too thick, you will find yourself rolling about trying to keep your balance, and since your aim is often to relax, you will be defeating your own purpose.

There are hundreds of variations of Yoga postures, enough to fill several books like this, so out of the many you should learn a group which will form a small balanced programme to which you can add according to choice. Most yogis finish up with a selection of favourite asanas which they find are enough to keep them in peak condition.

Now you must compose yourself for your session and many people find that the OM method is good for this purpose. OM, or Aum as it is sometimes spelt, is generally considered to be the sound of and for infinity. Your asanas are often a preliminary to meditation and so there is nothing out of place in sounding OM. It is sung usually as O-oo-mmmmm, or Ah-oo-mmmm. In either case you start with your mouth open and close it gradually until you are making a low humming through your closed lips. Repeat this sound three times.

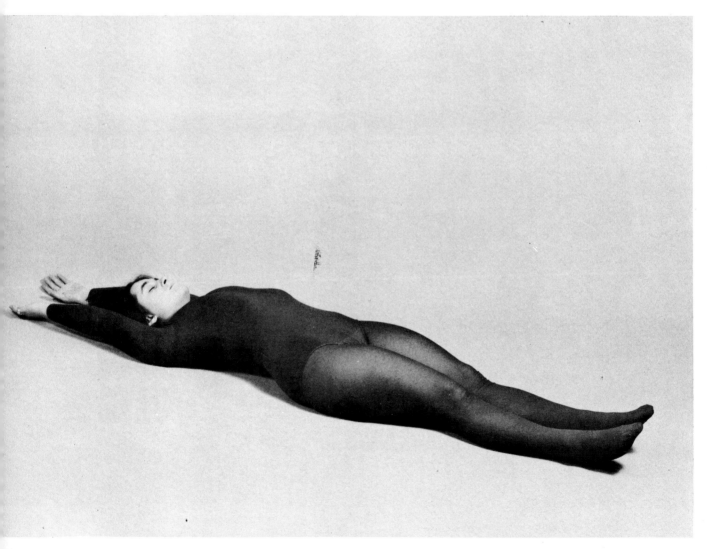

Its effect is to settle and clear your mind and to remind you that you are going to commit your whole concentration to the Yoga session before you. If you are in a situation where you feel that this unusual penetrating sound may be something of an embarrassment to you, then *think* the sound inside your head. Practise it out loud one day when you are alone and commit the sound of OM to memory. From that time on, you will be able to use it silently inside your mind. Eventually this can have as much effect as if you had used the sound out loud.

Janu Sirsasana, the **Alternate Leg Stretch**, is a good starting point for your session (see page 65). It is a simple stretch which anybody in any degree of stiffness can try. A stiff person will barely be able at first to make any movement, whereas an adept or a naturally supple person may be able to double up like a jackknife. The result doesn't matter. The important thing is that you are doing the posture at all.

Sit on the ground with your legs straight out in front of you. Draw in your left foot, using your hands, and tuck it as close to your body as you can manage. Preferably, your heel should touch your pelvic bone. Now raise your arms above your head and very slowly bend over to grasp your right foot. Your elbows go outwards and you lean over until your head touches your knee.

All right, so you can't reach either your foot or your ankle. Then simply grasp your leg just below the knee. Bend forward as far as you can manage *comfortably*. Hold for a count of five and then straighten up again. An alternative method for beginners is to use a twisted scarf. Hitch this over your foot and use it to pull yourself *gently* down. Do not try to stretch too far at first. Be content with only a small stretch and hold it for a short count. Do this three times; then change over and repeat with the other leg stretched out. You exhale as you bend over, but when you are holding the bent position you breathe naturally. Inhale as you come up.

This asana helps to tone up the liver and the digestion. It has a strong squeezing effect on the kidneys and this can be felt in the stretch of your back. You will probably find a startling improvement in the amount of stretch that you can manage even after only a week or two, but do not let it turn you into an end-gamer—someone on an achievement trip. As we said before, the important thing is to *do* the asana.

This head-to-knee position leads logically to the **Back Stretch** or **Paschimottanasana**. If you are a beginner, you can start this posture sitting up, but to gain the full benefit of the movement you should begin by lying flat on your back with your arms stretched out behind you.

Link your hands together and raise your arms up to a vertical position, above your head. Now you begin to raise your body off the floor and, as you do this, your hands are brought down towards your thighs. By the time you are sitting upright, your hands should be on the thighs. Continue the movement, leaning forward and sliding your hands down your legs as far as you can comfortably reach, as

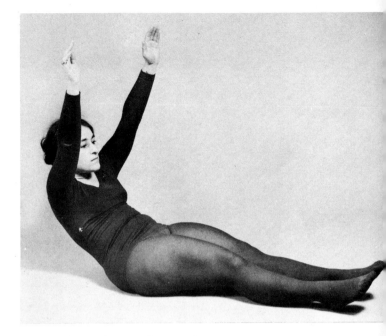

Keep your feet on the ground as you raise your arms.

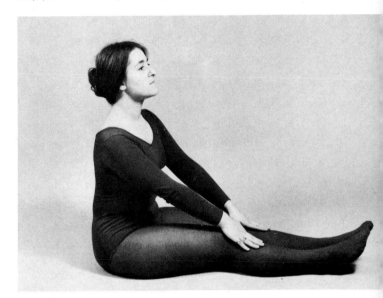

Slide your hands along your thighs.

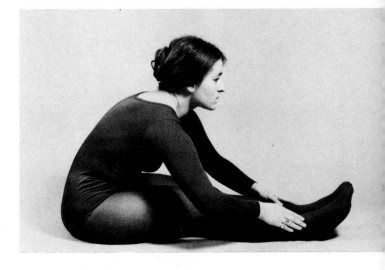

Reach only as far as is comfortable.

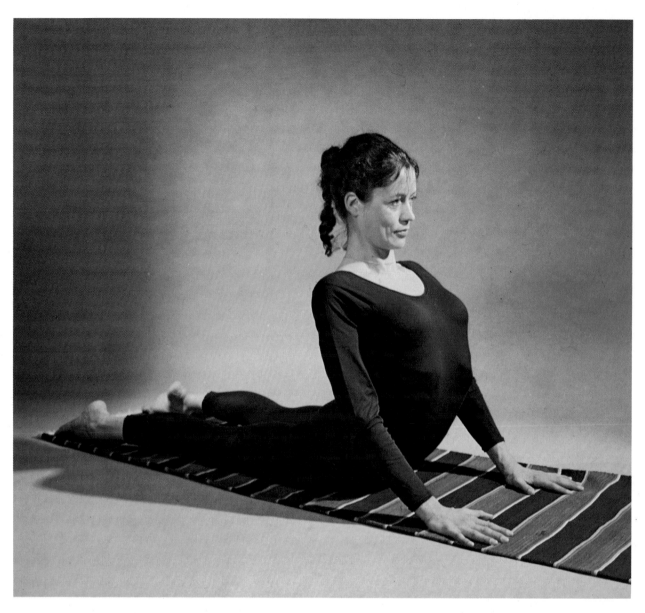

near to the feet as possible. Then try to bring your chest down toward your knees, keeping your elbows out. As with the Alternate Leg Stretch, you breathe out as you go forward, breathe naturally while you hold the position, and then inhale as you straighten up.

Once again, if you are stiff, begin by grasping your legs just below the knees. As your joints gradually loosen, so you will be able to reach further and further down your legs until you are holding your feet and completely doubled over. No matter how far you bend over, you should always be able to breathe comfortably. Keep your elbows out, your chest open, and your back flat or you will collapse your rib cage and make it difficult to breathe.

There is a basic rule in the practice of Yoga asanas which ensures that you develop evenly and gracefully. It is called the counter-pose rule. By this method, no one part of you can become over-developed in the way, for example, that some weight-lifters develop arms which are as thick as their legs. Yoga aims at a naturally balanced body, and a naturally balanced body is automatically graceful.

Above: A Cobra stretch as beautiful and complete as this will take years of practice.

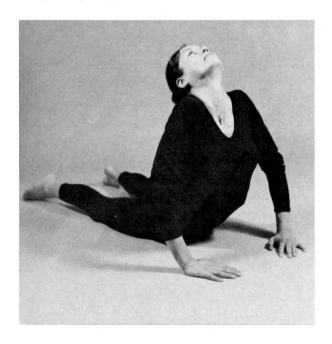

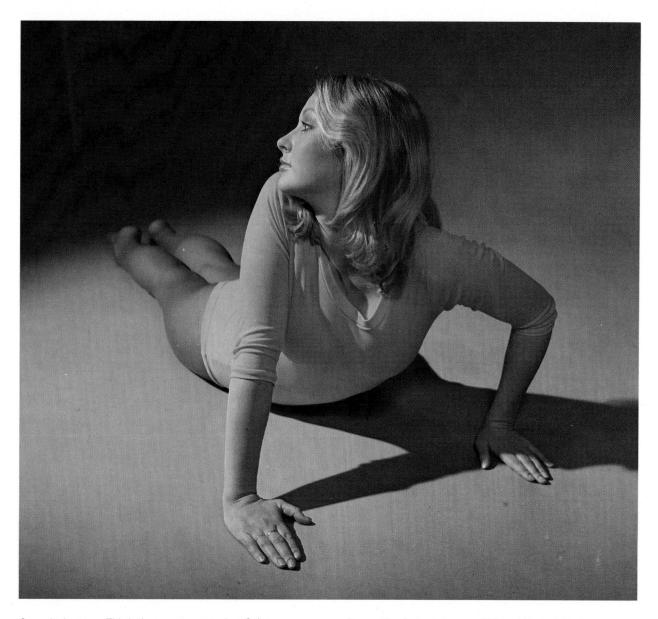

Opposite bottom: This is the wrong way to do a Cobra. See how the shoulders have come up round the ears.

Above: The Cobra is too easy? Then add a twist to it.

The counter-pose rule simply states that if you bend in one direction (and this applies particularly to the spine) then you must also bend in the opposite direction. Everything is always done symmetrically. The Janu Sirsasana is done always with first one leg tucked in and then the other. If you bend to the right for a posture, then you must bend to the left in the same posture. This does not mean that every movement must be instantly followed by its opposite, but it does mean that by the end of a session your spine should have spent as much time bending one way as the other.

Following this rule, it is logical after doing Paschimottanasana that you should perform a posture in which the spine is bent backwards instead of forwards. Therefore next on the list comes a completely traditional posture, known as **Bujanghasana,** the **Cobra.**

The Cobra is so named because its action is supposed to resemble that of a cobra raised ready to strike. Before you begin, it is very important to

realize that this asana is not the same as a Western 'push-up' exercise, whose aim is primarily to develop the shoulder and upper-arm muscles. The yogic Cobra is primarily a very powerful spinal stretch and it must be done very carefully if you want to gain the maximum benefit.

To perform it, you roll over and lie on your stomach. Turn your head to one side and relax with your hands by your sides. This preliminary relaxation is important. Next, you turn your head so that your nose is on the ground. Keep your knees together, extend your legs and keep your toes pointed. Now, bring your hands roughly level with your shoulders and pointing slightly inwards. Raise your head very slowly, then your neck, and then very gradually push your trunk off the floor. Feel the stretch gradually moving down your spine. Keep your thighs and buttocks tight so that your pelvis is pushed to the ground. Raise your eyes to look as high as possible and hold the position for a slow count of ten. Lower yourself at exactly the

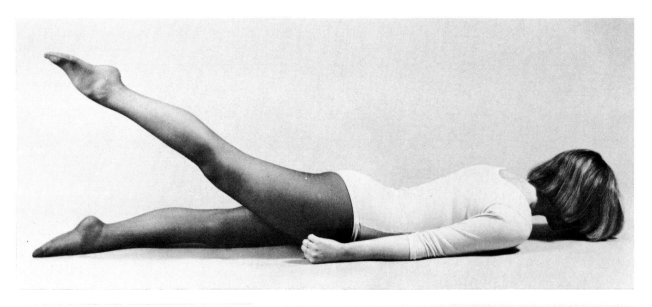

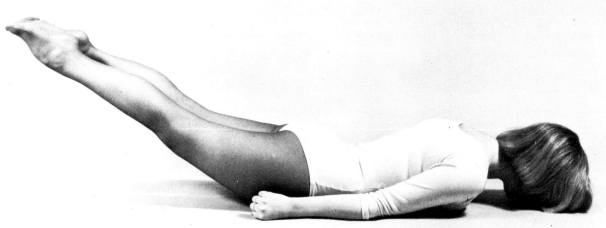

Above: Two versions of the Locust or Shalabasana.
Like many Yoga postures the full asana can be achieved
through several stages of increasing difficulty.
Opposite top: Holding the beginning of the Bow
Opposite bottom: For those who find this posture all too easy.
Rock backwards and forwards like a rocking horse.

same slow pace as you went up. None of this letting out a gasp of air and then flopping down to the ground. You do not relax until your head is safely resting on the ground turned to the side and your hands are back by your sides.

It is most important that you should raise yourself only a little at a time or you will not stretch your spine evenly. Spines are seldom uniformly stiff and if you raise yourself too quickly you may create a 'kink' in your spine at the point where it is most supple. The supple part will take all the movement and the stiff part will stay rigid. It may be months before the movement can be easily performed.

Take two breaths before you start to raise yourself. Breathe in as you go up, breathe naturally while you hold the position, and breathe out as you go down. Do the stretch about three times.

A few don'ts. Don't push up too quickly or too far. Don't sag so that your shoulders come up by your ears but keep your chest open and your shoulders down. Don't let your thigh muscles go slack so that you are dangling with nothing touching the ground between your hands and your knees. **Keep your hips and thighs** pressed to the ground.

Like the Janu Sirsasana, the posture stimulates the kidneys and internal organs. When you lie face down relaxed, you should be able to feel a warmth as the blood rushes again into the areas of your back which you have been contracting.

The Cobra is rated among the most important postures for the Westerner. Atrophied shoulder and back muscles, the result of continual stooping over machines and desks, receive tremendous exercise and an additional flow of blood. This blood also nourishes the nerve system which runs up and down the spine. Should these nerves lack their proper nourishment, then almost every single functional part of our organism is affected and in time disorders will inevitably arise.

During the time that you hold the position, your breathing creates an internal motion which has the effect of massaging the liver and the other digestive organs. The Cobra is often recommended for the treatment of slipped discs, but great care should be observed over this and medical advice obtained. Much depends on the direction in which the vertebral disc has slipped; in some circumstances the Cobra can be quite unsuitable.

The leverage on your spine is very strong in this pose. Consequently, it is at the same time very beneficial if handled properly and damaging if handled badly. If you feel pain, just cut short the exercise and practise more gently next time. Follow the rule of listening to what your body tells you and you will come to no harm. Any pain that arises will tell you either that you are going too far or that this movement is not suitable. You will only get into trouble if you try to show off to, or compete with, yourself.

Shalabasana or the **Locust Pose** usually follows the Cobra because it also works on the spine but starting at the opposite end, the bottom end. The Locust is an extremely active posture and it is certainly no posture for meditation. Indeed even adepts can seldom hold the full position for very long, and it requires considerable strength just to reach it. Nevertheless it is a very suitable posture for beginners because it can be graded so that it becomes really quite easy to do. Even in a modified form it is excellent for tightening up the muscles around the hips and the stomach.

Here, then, is an elementary form of Locust. Lie face down with the ball of the chin firmly on the ground. Place your fists (thumbs downwards) firmly on the floor by your sides. Press hard down with your chin and your fists, and slowly raise your left leg as high as you can behind you. Hold for a count of five and lower the leg slowly. Repeat the process with the other leg.

There is a little more to the exercise than this. You should press down harder with the hand on the same side as the leg which is being raised. And you should keep both hips touching the floor; this makes the exercise much more difficult to do, but it gives more benefit than raising the leg higher by twisting the hips. Do not allow your leg to bend. Most of the raising should be done by the muscles in the small of your back.

It may require weeks or even months of raising one leg at a time before you are strong enough to try the complete Locust, raising both legs at the same time. This is far from easy, so do not strain yourself trying to do the posture. You must have enough strength to raise and lower yourself slowly, and you should always come down under control and not just collapse. Even an adept will not expect to hold the position for much more than a slow count of ten. As it is a very strenuous posture you will need a short relaxation after it in order to allow your breathing to return to normal. The full Locust is seldom repeated more than three times.

The effect of the Locust is similar to that of the Cobra in that there is a very strong action in the area of the kidneys. The nervous system in the spine is stimulated, as are the digestive organs. The most important effect is probably the strengthening of the muscles in the sacral area at the bottom of the spine. This is the area that must become flexible and strong if you are to gain full control over your posture and avoid the slipped disc which can result from the slightest inopportune movement if the back muscles have been allowed to deteriorate through lack of use. As one fashionable osteopath

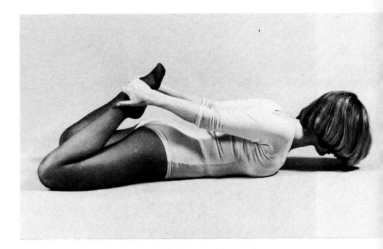

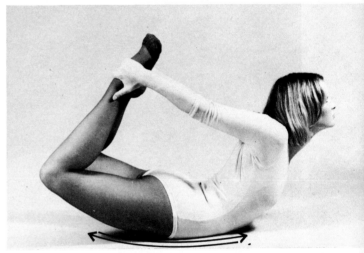

put it, 'I just never get people among my patients who have an active outdoor job; after fifteen years this has gone long past the point of coincidence.'

It's such an old story: 'There I was—one minute I was perfectly alright, and then all I did was bend over, and I couldn't move. It was agony.' Every spine is at risk almost every minute of the day, even while simply sitting in a chair, but the risk is quite negligible so long as the spine is supported by muscle which has been kept in good condition and is supple enough to allow us to carry out the various activities we attempt. A healthy spine is a key to well-being and it is no accident that the action of the spine forms the very core of so many Yoga postures.

Dhanurasana, the **Bow Pose**, is often used to complete a sequence of postures which contains the Cobra and the Locust. At first sight it would simply seem to combine their effects, but in fact this is not so. In both the Cobra and the Locust the back muscles are under strong contraction and do most of the work. In the Bow they are largely inactive.

The Bow is usually practised after the Locust and is begun by lying face down and concentrating on relaxing the back. The first movement is to exhale and grasp the ankles with the hands, the right hand to the right ankle, the left hand to the left ankle. Take two breaths and ensure that the grasp is comfortable. Now exhale and pull the knees and the chest off the floor. They should rise equally

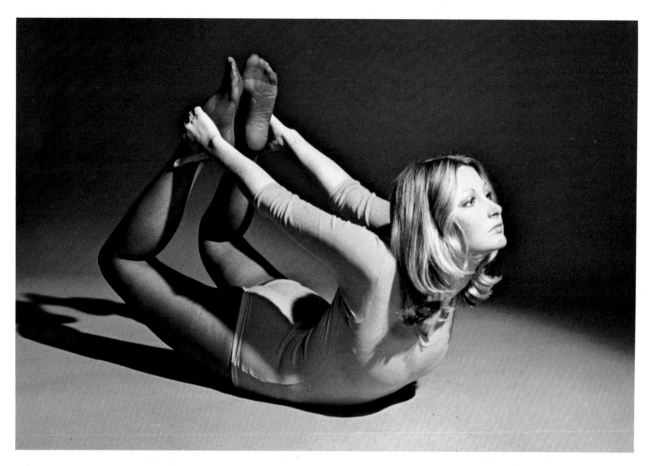

The completed Bow or Dhanurasana

so that you are balanced. Once the preliminary rise is made, the upward pull is created by the legs. If you try to straighten the legs, you will automatically pull the chest upwards. You do not draw the bow by contracting the muscles in the centre of your back; you draw it by pulling on your arms with your legs, the "bowstring". Try to maintain a balance. Your knees and your chin should always be at roughly the same level, however high you manage to draw yourself. The importance of this becomes clear when you consider moving onto the second part of the Bow, which is a dynamic movement.

In the first part of the movement, you raise yourself so that you are balanced on your stomach, not on your ribs or your pelvis. Once in this position you breathe naturally (though possibly a little fast owing to the general stress). Hold the position for half a minute to a minute. Then relax and slowly come down to a prone position. Let go of your ankles, straighten the legs, and relax.

The dynamic part of the Bow follows from the raised position. When you are able to assume this position easily, and only then, you begin to rock yourself gently backwards and forwards like a rocking horse, gradually increasing the movement until your knees touch the ground on the backward rock and your chin on the forward rock. Do not carry on until you are exhausted: do it only two or three times at first. Increase the rocking movement only when you are able to maintain complete control. When you have finished the rocking, you should still be able to lower yourself gradually to the ground.

An even more ambitious version of the Bow includes rolling sideways while holding the bow position. In all of these positions and variations the breath can be operated as follows:

1. inhale when the head rises and exhale when you lower it;
2. breathe normally throughout; or
3. hold the breath with the lungs full – this is not recommended except for adepts.

It is important to keep this posture symmetrical, and this is achieved by making sure that the ankles remain in contact with each other. The knees can be allowed to separate, but if the ankles part then you may pull one leg up higher than the other.

The effect of the posture, especially if the rocking version is used, is to tone up the viscera and the pancreas and to stretch the nerves and muscles of the spinal column. It is especially helpful after long days at desks or benches. There is also a general stimulation of the breathing and circulation, resulting from the massage of the solar plexus when the whole of the body is balanced on it. Naturally this asana is never attempted on a full stomach.

TWISTING THE SPINE

Your spine is capable of an enormous range of movement and your programme of Yoga asanas would be failing if it did not supply exercises to increase this potential. So far we have bent the spine backwards and forwards and sideways, so it only remains to supply methods of twisting it either way. The commonest and most famous posture for this purpose is known as **Ardha Matsyendrasana**, and unlike most Yoga postures it is not named after the action of an animal but after the yogi who was reputed to have invented it, Matsyendrasana. 'Ardha' means 'half', and it is the **Half Twist** that is most usually used, because the full posture needs such suppleness that very few yogis include it in their daily programme.

Even the half-twist is more than many people can manage at first. But a simple path of development has been devised so that you can start with very little effort and gradually build up to the complete posture, which is surprisingly comfortable once you are into it. Just keep in your mind the fact that the top half of your body will be moving in the opposite direction to the bottom half. There is also a bound version in which you can hold yourself well enough to meditate if you wish.

To start, try the simplest of possible twists. Sit on the ground with your legs straight out in front of you. Now twist your body to the right and place your hands on the ground at your right. Do this to the left as well (see page 76).

The next step is to return to your original sitting position, grasp your right leg, and lift it over your left. Your right foot should be just below and beside the left knee, which makes a very slight twist. Now you do what you did the first time: twist your body to the right and, if you can, place your hands on the ground. If you cannot, there is an alternative position. Having twisted to the right, you slide your left arm over your raised knee and grasp the other knee. Your other arm you place on the ground behind you. Turn your head to the right, away from your feet (see page 76).

It is important to understand that the back of your left elbow presses against your raised knee, because this increases the twist by pressing your knee further over. As you loosen up, so you move your leg further in until your foot is about opposite your knee. Now you are ready to try the **Completed Half Twist** (see page 77 and 78).

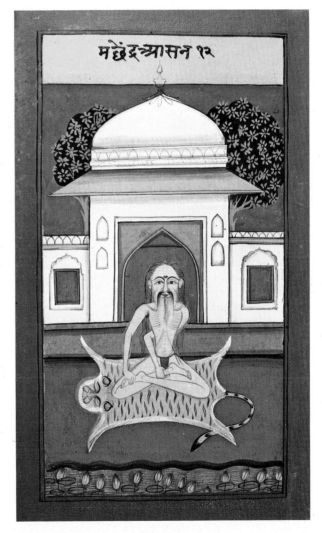

When yogis appear in art they show a continuity of Yoga technique extending over thousands of years. This is from an eighteenth-century Yoga album from the Punjab.

Sit with your legs straight out. Draw the left foot in with your hands and tuck it under your pelvis. Now take your right foot and lift your right leg over the left so that the right foot is as far back as you can manage and still have it on the ground. The shin should be as nearly vertical as you can make it. Now twist your body to the right and slide the back of the left elbow over the raised knee. If the knee is high enough, you may find that it will be your shoulder that you have to get over your knee.

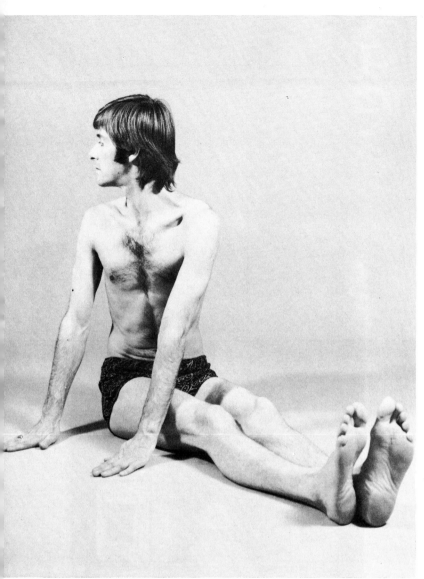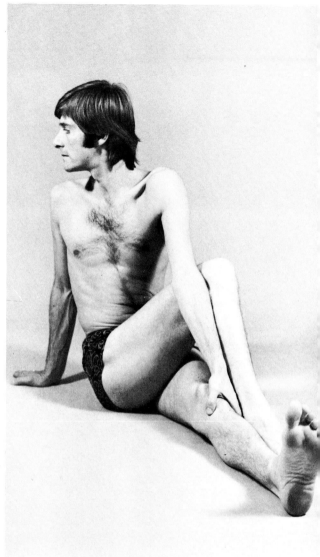

Grasp your left knee with your left hand. Take your right hand as far round behind your back as you can manage and turn your head to the right.

In this position the stomach and the diaphragm are naturally slightly squeezed, so you may find that your breathing has to be shallow, but keep it as quiet and even as you can.

When you have held the posture for as long as you find comfortable, slowly unwind, sit straight and breathe slowly and deeply. Then perform the twist turning in the opposite direction. A couple of repetitions either way is usually enough. If you want to remain a long time in the posture then you should use the bound version. The difference is that you push your arm through the arch of the leg and join your hands behind your back. The whole posture is then locked in place comfortably for as long as you want to stay that way. Physically there is no particular advantage in remaining in one position for a very long time, but the Complete Twist can be used as a meditational posture.

The **Standing Twist** is a very simple twisting posture. Raise your arms above your head and link the thumbs together. Breathe out, twisting the upper part of your body to the right. Then slowly twist to the front while breathing in. Take care not to twist your hips too much or this will reduce the twist on the spine. The linking of the movement to the breath makes it very effective. Again, of course, you should twist both ways, left and right, an equal number of times.

In these last two chapters you have a complete set of asanas to flex the spine in every direction. They are the fundamental asanas for Hatha Yoga. There are many more and variations on variations (catering for every conceivable need or variety of physique) but basically for any person in more or less normal health the asanas given here can ensure a rise to peak condition.

Once more, bear in mind that Yoga asanas are not meant to be muscle-builders. They are health builders. They work on the nerves, the endocrine system, and the circulation.

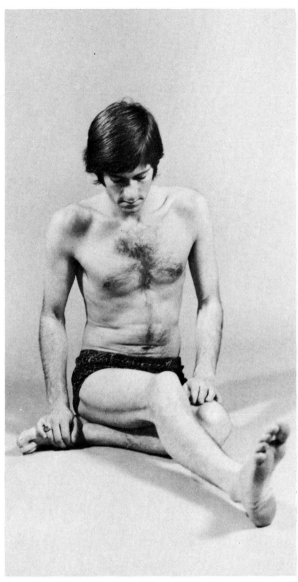

Opposite: Two very simple twists
Left and below: The first three stages in Ardha Matsyendrasana
The original version of the Matsyendrasana proved so difficult that it has fallen largely into disuse and the modified version, or Ardha Matsyendrasana, is commonly used. In the original, the foot comes over the thigh as in a Lotus. The true identity of Matsyendra is something of an enigma. He was not an Indian, his Sanskrit was poor, and it was not the language he used for teaching. It seems that his natural tongue was Aramaic, the same language as was used by Jesus of Nazareth. There is a school of thought which claims that in fact he may actually have been Jesus of Nazareth. Of course the records of those times are so sparse that it is impossible to be accurate even within half a century, but Matsyendra and Jesus of Nazareth could conceivably have existed around the same period. However, evidence agrees that certainly somebody was crucified in the name of Jesus of Nazareth, while the records elsewhere are equally certain that Matsyendra lived on to a ripe old age, leaving a small family behind him. It may be no more than a coincidence that Matsyendra adopted his yogic name from that of Vishnu's first incarnation, while the original sign of the early Christians was also—a fish.

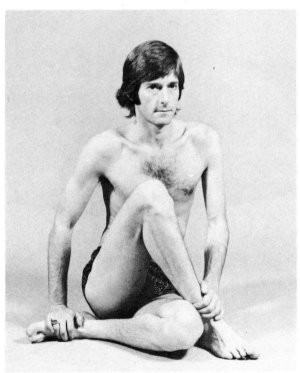

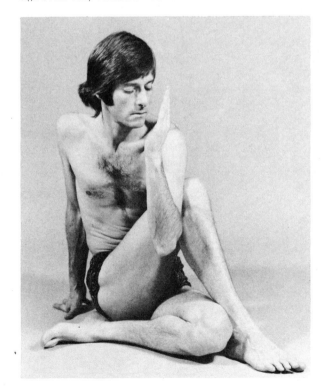

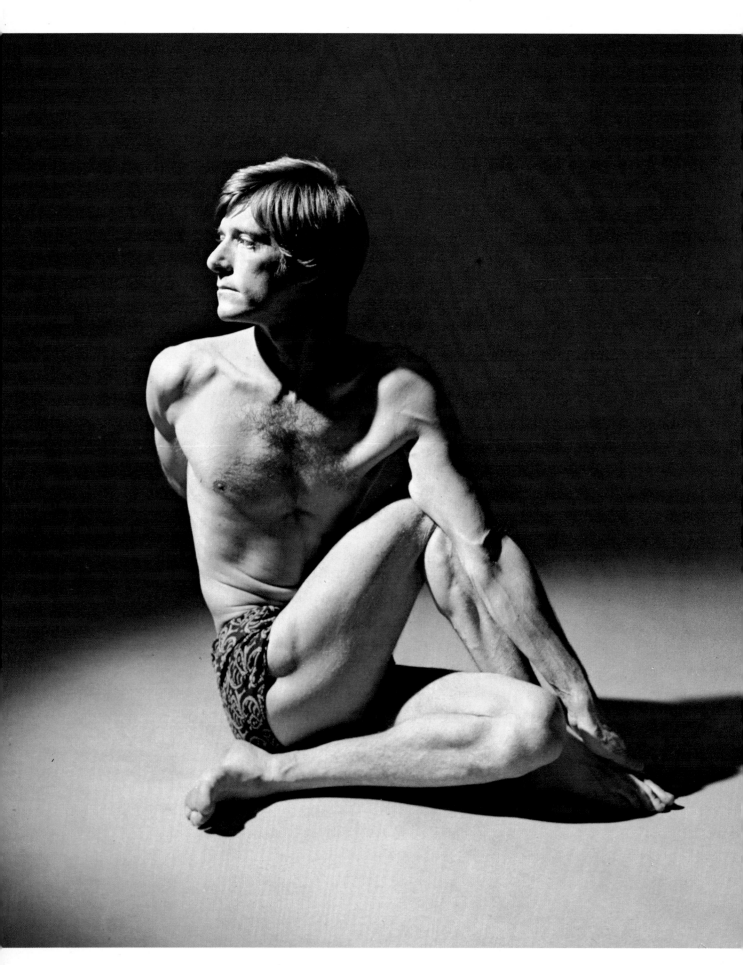

Ardha Matsyendrasana completed

YOGA'S UPSIDE-DOWN ROUTE TO HEALTH

Everyone who has ever practised Yoga for any length of time groans inwardly whenever they hear one of those hoary old jokes about standing on your head. 'You do Yoga? Ha, ha! Well, stand on your head. Go on, let's see you!' As Yogi Bhajan said, 'If that was all there was to Yoga, then all the best yogis would be in circuses.'

There are some yogis who have never stood on their heads in their lives: standing on one's head is not a pastime suited to everybody's physique. Nevertheless, it is an undoubted fact that yogis do tend to turn themselves upside down occasionally, with good reason and with good effect. If this upside-down business is examined objectively, it turns out to be less eccentric than at first appears.

The whole of Yoga is based on the idea of making use of natural laws and not trying to oppose them. In the upside-down postures of Yoga, the yogi makes use of the well-known law of gravity. Think of the expressions 'Oh, that gets me down!' and 'I feel dragged down with tiredness.' Both illustrate the effect of gravity on the sensations of the human being. If you examine the face or body of an old person, you will see very readily how gravity has taken its toll. Jowls do not float upwards: they hang down, pulled that way by gravity. Breasts sag, so do jawlines; legs become varicose, overfilled with blood dragged down by gravity. Almost every sign of old age can be traced to the effect of gravity.

Nobody knows any longer which particular yogi it was who sat down and produced the obvious idea that if gravity drags you down into old age, then by reversing gravity, you ought to reverse the ageing process as well. But turn yourself upside down, and this—to a quite surprising degree—is what can happen. Of course, if you think objectively about it, then it is so very obvious.

Deterioration of the human body generally arises from two things, starvation and stagnation. If the tissues do not receive enough food they starve. Starvation can occur because you are not eating enough, because you are not eating correctly, or because you are not doing enough exercise to make the blood flow thoroughly into all parts of your body. Stagnation also results from sluggish circulation. The blood which brings the nourishment to your body also washes away the waste products. It's like the milkman who delivers fresh milk on the way in and takes away the empties on his way out.

If you are always one way up, with your head up

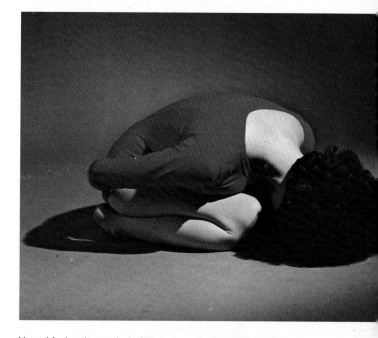

Yoga Mudra, the symbol of Yoga, can also be used purely physically to lift the internal organs; the legs are crossed in the Lotus and the fists placed at the base of the abdomen.

and your feet down, then blood will always tend to drain toward your feet and away from your head. Your circulation is designed to work so that plenty of blood will go to your head, but this does not alter the fact that if your head is up the blood will drain away from it. If you are always that way up, then the liquid in your lungs will always tend to drain down into the bottom of your lungs, where it can form a stagnant pool which quickly gives rise to infections.

But turn your body upside down, even if it is only for a short period of time, and you are freed from that persistent pull of gravity which draws you daily lower into age. The unwanted blood will drain out of the legs, where it has been building the potential for varicose veins, and into the head, which needs the biggest and best supply it can get if you are going to remain quick-witted and intelligent through your middle years and into old age. As a matter of fact, even a short session upside down is sufficient to get your mind moving again in the middle of a tiring day.

Long before the notorious Headstand came into use, there were other upside-down postures for

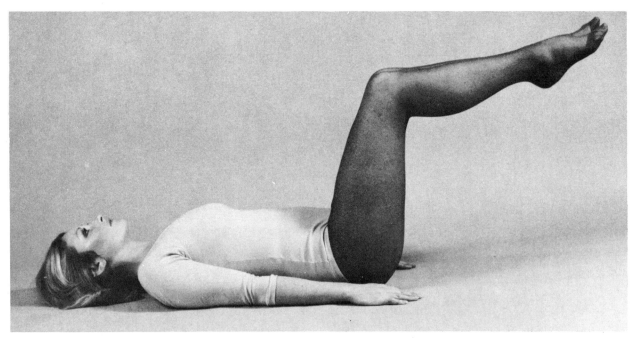

yogis. These are much easier and safer than the Headstand and they are used everywhere in Yoga to this very day. Probably the best known is Sarvangasana but Viparita Karani is nearly as well known. The most noticeable difference between these two and the Headstand is that they hold the spine under much less compression. Almost anyone can manage either of them and, though their effect differs slightly from that of the Headstand, the similarity is so close that for most practical purposes they can replace it, that is assuming that one or two other routine postures are used, such as the Pose of a Child, Pada Hastasana, or Yoga Mudra.

There is another reason why the yogis regard these upside-down postures as so especially helpful. The explanation hovers on the borderlines between bio-physics and metaphysics. Both Western scientists and yogis recognize that there are certain force currents that flow between the outer atmosphere and the earth. The nature and extent of these currents is not yet wholly known but the yogis have long operated a rule-of-thumb approach. Thus, if you turn the body upside-down, you not only reverse the effect of gravity, but you also reverse the flow of the force currents from the earth through the body and with an apparently equally beneficial effect, the theory being that a 're-balancing' process takes place. Undeniably most people seem to find it a tranquillizing experience. One teacher, B.K.S. Iyengar, frequently places highly nervous pupils in upside-down positions for very considerable periods. The interesting thing is that, unlike tranquillizing by drugs, the use of the upside-down postures does not produce a blurred consciousness. The brain seems to become both tranquillized and at the same time clarified.

The start of both Viparita Karani and the Shoulder Stand is the same but the end positions are subtly and importantly different. To begin **Viparita Karani**, otherwise known as the **Whole Body Posture**, the **Half Shoulder** or **Half Candle**, you lie on your back on the floor with

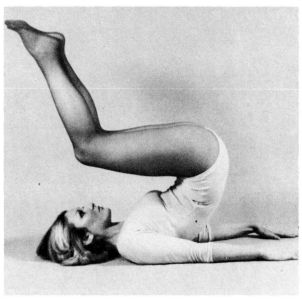

The first three stages of Viparita Karani, Savangasana, and Halasana are the same. Anyone whose back is strong enough should carry out these actions with the legs held straight.

your hands palms down by your sides. Slowly raise the legs, vertical and then press down with the hands while bringing the legs forward until they are above your head. This will have the effect of pulling your hips up from the floor. Move first one hand and then the other from the floor to your hips so that your body is supported by your hands under your hips. The head, shoulders, and back of the arms down to the elbows form the base on which you are balanced. Your legs should be straight and your feet should be roughly above your head (see page 82). To come down, you put your hands on the ground and lower yourself very slowly.

There is a school of thought which dictates that the legs should be vertical above the hips but this is somewhat more difficult to hold for any length of time. Keep the chest well open so that you can breathe properly. Do not allow yourself to collapse

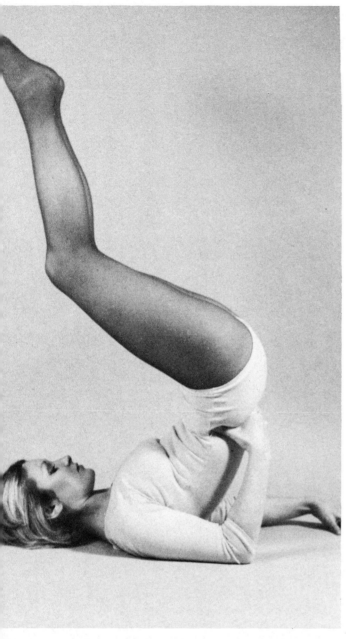

sexual energy, is burnt, lost or exhausted by the internal fire or sun element in the body. This is a natural process which takes place in everyone, the result being old age and dissipation. With the prolonged and constant practice of Viparita Karani Mudra, the flow and the process can be reversed, causing the sexual energy to flow up to Vishuddhi Chakra and unite with the nectar. The process is called the sublimation of sexual energy, the result being a re-vitalisation and rejuvenation of the entire body and mind.'

You can begin by holding this position for thirty seconds, then gradually increasing the period to thirty minutes. While you hold it, the mind should be concentrated on the vishuddi cakra, which is a point roughly at the thyroid gland in the throat. But it is not worth bothering about that until you have managed to balance yourself reasonably comfortably and safely in the basic position. It serves little purpose to attempt to concentrate on the cakra if your mind is continually having to dart away in order to check your body position.

Sarvangasana, the **Shoulder Stand**, is sometimes also known as the **Shoulder Balance**. This posture is considered to be second only to the Headstand in the strength of its effect. You begin as before, lying flat on your back with the palms of your hands pressing on the ground. Exhale and then slowly raise your legs until your hips have been lifted off the ground, only this time bring your legs further over your head so that your body is in a more vertical position. Place your hands so they support the back of the rib cage. Now raise your legs so that the whole of your body and your legs are as nearly vertical to the ground as you can manage (see page 82). You may want to remain in this position a while so be sure that your shoulders are back and your chest held open. Then you will have plenty of room to breathe naturally. Begin by maintaining the position for half a minute and gradually increase to thirty minutes.

This is a relatively easy pose to do, but the most common error seems to be in getting it lopsided. Be sure that you come up straight, that your arms are both at the same angle and that your hands are symmetrically placed in the back of your ribs. Often you can improve on your position after half a minute. As the body becomes accustomed to the posture it is possible to ease your hands further away from your hips and toward your shoulders and this helps to bring the whole of your body vertical.

When you are in the full position it should require virtually no strength at all to keep you there. The whole of your body and legs should be completely relaxed. To ensure that your legs are properly relaxed, you should not point the toes (although it may look more elegant) but allow the feet to assume their most natural position. You can aid this relaxation by learning to shake the muscles until you are sure that there is no build-up of tension. When you are fully relaxed, your leg muscles will begin to "creep downwards" and "shrink" as the unneeded tension and surplus blood are drained away from them.

or your ribs will be held tight. Think of yourself as being in three straight lines: a short one, along the floor from the tip of your head to your shoulders; a longer one formed by the part of your body propped up by your hands at an angle of roughly 45° to the ground; and finally the longest one, a straight line upwards from your hips to bring your feet over your head. Unlike the Shoulder Stand, your chin should not be pressed against the top of your ribs. This creates the important difference between the two postures. In Viparita Karani the blood flows more freely up to the brain and does not create a build-up at the thyroid gland.

Swami Satyananda gives the following yogic explanation of the effects of this upside-down posture:

'There is a nectar which flows from the Vishuddhi Chakra, the throat or thyroid centre, down to the Manipura Chakra, the Solar Plexus or centre of solar energy. This nectar upon uniting with the

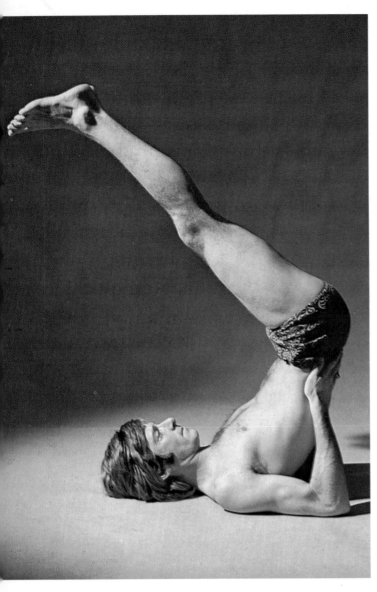

Viparita Karani completed

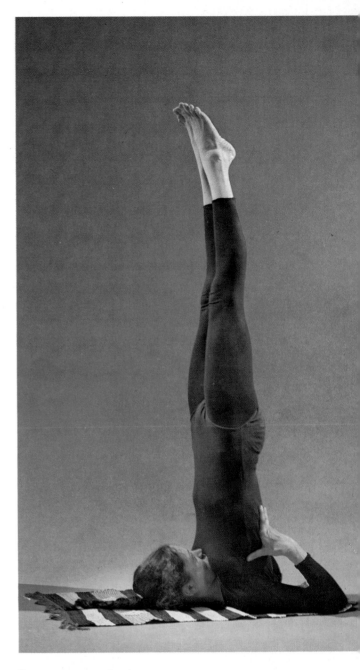

Savangasana completed

It is important to try to place the chin in the notch at the top of the ribs so that it forms the "lock" which creates the build-up of blood around the thyroid gland. Do this by bringing the *ribs to the chin* and *not* the chin to the ribs. Bringing the chin to the ribs will tend to pull the whole posture downwards and create tension and a collapsed-lung position. Bringing the ribs to the chin will help to expand the chest and bring the body into a balanced position on the shoulders in which you can relax totally, since no muscle effort will be needed to hold you upright.

People with a weak lower-back may find difficulty in raising themselves into this position slowly and gracefully, and so there is a simple alternative method for beginners. Instead of the legs being straight when raised off the floor, you bend the knees and bring the legs over your head bent. If even this is difficult, a rolled towel can be placed beneath the hips so that it creates a seesaw of the torso, and with this and a bent knee even the most out-of-breath and obese persons can turn themselves upside down. Coming down again the over-

weight beginner need only roll down into a ball and then gradually unwind.

The benefits of the Shoulder Stand are similar to those of Viparita Karani and the Headstand. Basically it is the reversal of gravity and the force currents. The legs and lower organs of the body are decongested. The lungs can be drained, although it should be recognized that at first this may seem to aggravate any respiratory condition. Nevertheless, deep breathing in Sarvangasana can be a preliminary stage in the removal of bronchial congestion and is sometimes used in treating asthma. There is, of course, an increased flow of blood to the brain in this posture and, because of the chin lock, a big boost to the thyroid gland. Because of the latter, the posture is not advisable for anyone who suffers from hyperthyroid problems since it would stimulate an already excessive out-put. Other than this there are

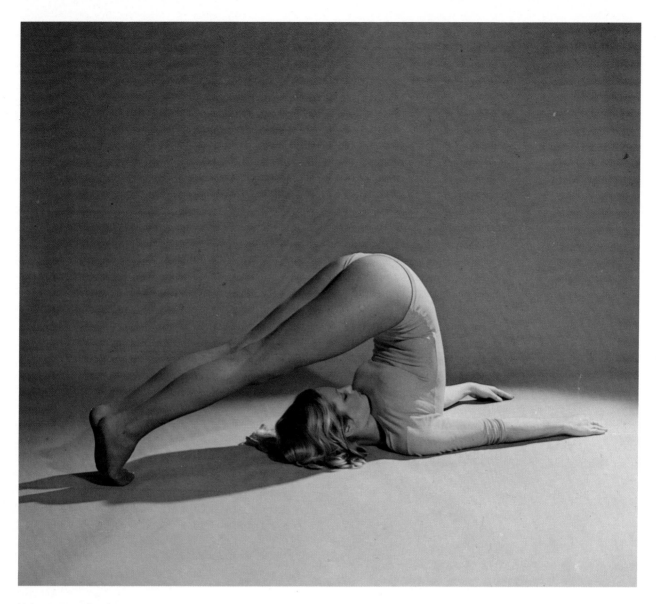

Halasana completed

few contra-indications. It is not advised for those with angina, scelerosis of the brain, or sinusitis.

Since the Shoulder Stand is such a remarkable revitalizer, it can be used at brief intervals throughout the day and indeed is better used in this way than for a long period at one single session. It is especially suitable for people who may be developing varicose veins from long hours of standing.

Sarvangasana is usually followed by Halasana, but if it is not it should always be followed by a counter pose which will stretch the neck in the opposite direction. The pose generally used for this is Matsyasana, which will be explained on page 84.

Halasana, the **Plough**, can be started on its own, or it can follow naturally after the Shoulder Stand. It is in some ways better to do it after the Shoulder Stand because there is less likelihood of going over into a collapsed position which will hinder breathing. Follow the directions for the Shoulder Stand, but in this case, instead of bringing the legs to a vertical position, the hands remain on the floor and you continue the forward action of the legs until they touch the ground behind your head. This is a

very simple movement to achieve but it can easily lead to injuries.

The most important thing is not to rush the process of getting the feet down to the floor. It can take literally months, especially if you have an overweight problem. The Plough stretches the spine very considerably and the key to doing it easily lies in suppleness in the lower part of the spine and in the thighs. If you attempt to force the feet down to the ground while this part of the body is too stiff, you will transfer considerable strain to the neck and may easily pull a neck or shoulder muscle. At first be content simply to let your legs dangle off the ground. Gradually, over a period of weeks or possibly even longer, they will sink down. If you want to remain in the Plough and find that dangling is too tiring, then the legs can be rested on some books or the seat of a chair to take the strain out of the position.

If you are starting the Plough from the Shoulder Stand position, you should feel no great increase of tension in the neck and shoulders. The stretch should take place further down in the spine and in

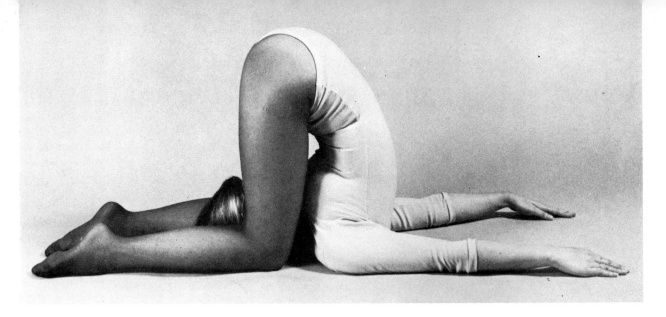

Many people use Karna Peethasana *(above)* as a comfortable halfway house when ending the Plough.

the thighs. You should have the feeling as you slowly lower your legs toward the ground that your spine is unwinding.

In the Plough, as in the Shoulder Stand, it is important to be sure that the pose is not performed in a lopsided way. Your legs should go straight over and be directly in line behind the head. To come out of the Plough, you simply bend your legs, part them so that they pass either side of your head, and, while keeping your head and shoulders on the floor, slowly unroll until you are lying out flat on your back.

For a beginner, the posture should be maintained for only a short period and it is a good idea to perform the movement two or three times, holding for a slow count of ten. Unless under the personal tuition of a yogi, this pose is seldom held for more than five minutes at a time but there is no reason, if the pupil is well advanced, for it not to be held for much longer.

There are two advanced starting positions for the Plough which can be used if you do not want to tag the Plough onto the Shoulder Stand. The first is to lie on the ground with your hands stretched out behind your head and to lift the legs quite straight and very slowly over the head until they touch the ground. For the more advanced student the pose can be started by placing the hands on the top of the head or just under the back of the head. In both of these cases, it is important to make sure that the spine is as flat as possible and that the neck is stretched before you start, but neither should be attempted unless you can already do the Plough easily in its standard form.

During the pose, your mind should be directed to whichever body area you are moving until you reach the point where you remain completely still. Then the concentration should be in the thyroid area. It can be moved to the solar plexus if you want to do some deep breathing. It is most important to concentrate on performing the action very slowly, smoothly and gracefully. A well-performed Plough can be a most elegant demonstration of the qualities that can be developed by Yoga.

The Plough is another of the tonic/tranquillizer postures. It is a strong stimulant to the thyroid gland and to the entire spinal column, which is stretched evenly from one end to the other. In order to be sure that this stretch is carried out evenly, the movements must be done very slowly so that each vertebral joint in the spine is moved separately. Any attempt to hurry the process will simply place the burden of moving fastest and most on the joint which is already the most supple and probably also the weakest, an effect which has already been noted in the Cobra.

Almost all of the life mechanism inside the torso is stimulated in the Plough posture and there are few contra-indications, these being confined to hernias, the beginning of menstruation and the later stages of pregnancy, when of course the increased size of the abdomen makes it difficult to lower the legs to the ground.

The last three postures have in common the strong stretching of the spine in one direction and all of them must be followed by a counter pose so that the spinal column is brought back to a normal balance. Fortunately this can be achieved in much less time. In all three postures the chin has been pressed to the chest and the expansion of the thorax has been prevented. **Matsyasana**, the **Fish Pose**, arches the neck, frees its movement, and removes the compression from the thyroid gland. It allows the abdomen, which has been constricted, to expand and is an excellent posture for assisting the development of the deep breathing which empties the bottom of the lungs. It is very often used to teach beginners who breathe only with the upper part of chest how to breathe abdominally. When the Fish posture is performed, the upper part of the chest is held almost immobile so that it is automatically only practical to breathe abdominally.

You begin by sitting up from the lying position in which you ended the Plough or the Shoulder Stand. Your legs are straight out in front of you. Lean backwards and put first one elbow on the ground, then the other. Lean back onto the elbows and arch the back. Then drop the head back so that if possible the crown of the head is on the floor and you are looking along the floor upside down.

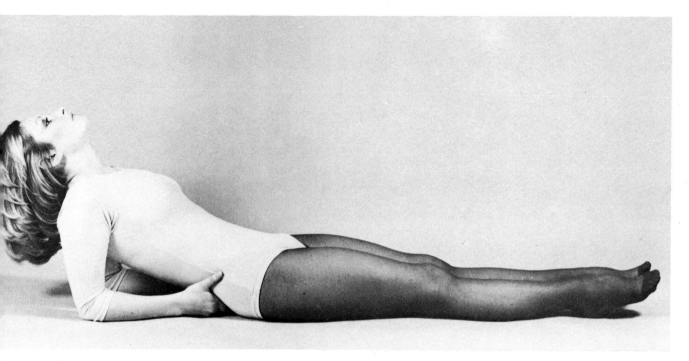

Matsyasana, counterpose to Savangasana, in two stages. It should be held for one third the time spent in Savangasana.

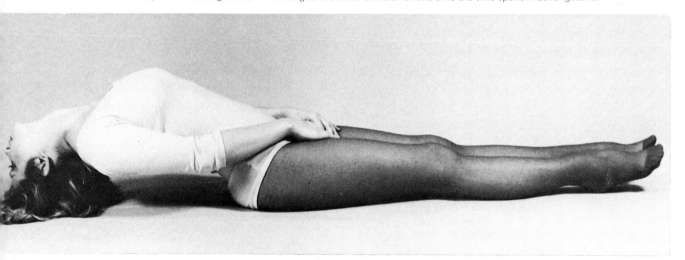

So far, your weight has been resting on your elbows. Now arch your back and brace your neck so that you can remove your elbows from the ground and rest your hands on your thighs. The body is now in an arch, supported at one end by the crown of the head and at the other by the buttocks. The posture is held for a slow count of ten. This time is seldom increased to more than five minutes.

The Fish can be performed from a kneeling position (Vajrasana) or from a cross-legged position (Sukhasana or Padmasana, the classic Lotus Seat). The ultimate aim is to be able to lean backwards, place the head on the ground, hold, and then sit up again without using the elbows at all. This requires very considerable strength and suppleness but the really important part is not the demonstration of finesse but the final position: elegance is secondary.

The real importance of Matsyasana lies in the stretching of the chest and strengthening of the back. It acts directly on round shoulders. We have become so accustomed to living with hunched shoulders that many people find the Fish position surprisingly difficult, and the ability to drop the head back far enough may take some time. Once the opening up begins to take place, an actual change in the physical measurements of the ribs is not at all unusual. This of course leads in turn to an increased lung capacity, which again permits a boost to the whole organism. The Fish also stimulates the adrenal and genital glands, and the abdominal breathing creates a natural massage for all the organs in the lower part of the torso.

The Fish is one of the classical postures of Yoga and taken in combination with the previous postures it covers a great deal of ground. Anybody who uses the upside-down postures and the Fish is stimulating and stretching almost everything in the human body that there is to be both stimulated and stretched.

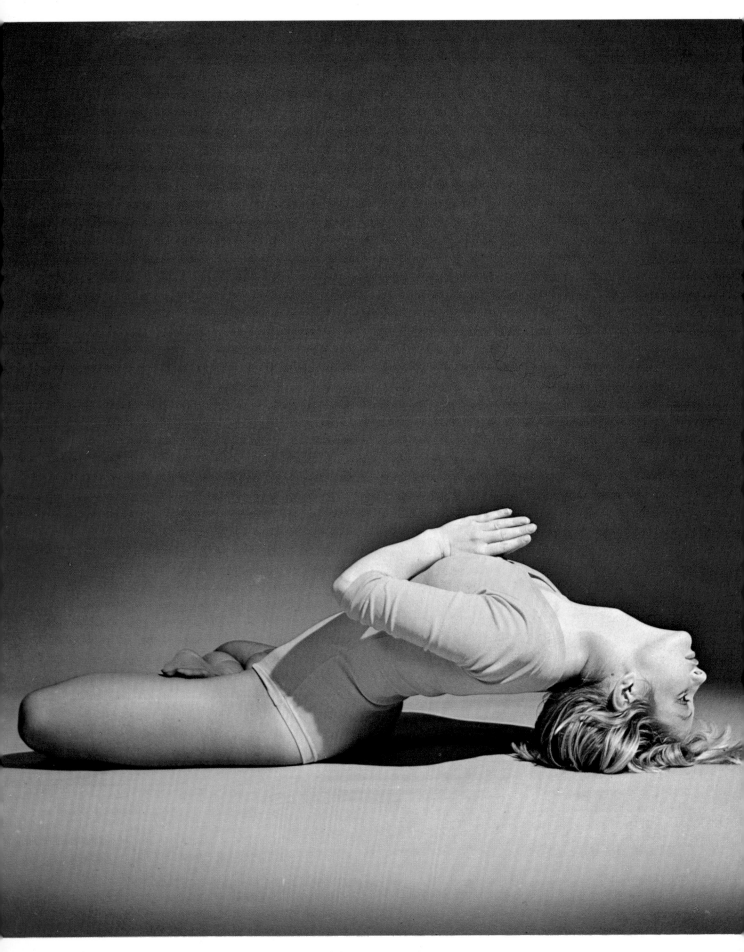

In the traditional form of Matsyasana, the Fish Pose, the legs are in a cross-legged position.

The KING OF THE ASANAS

No description of the upside-down postures of Yoga would be complete without the **Sirshasana**, the **Headstand**, known to yogis the world over as King of the Asanas because of the tremendously strong effect that it has on virtually the entire body. Naturally the very acrobatic nature of the posture is attractive–it sets the person who can do it a little bit above the run of the mill–and it is inevitable that more people will attempt the Headstand than should, strictly speaking.

Your shoulders and neck should have had not less than six months' special exercise so that they are ready to take your weight. And there are several other provisos about the use of the Headstand. Do not attempt it if you have:

1. a high blood-pressure,
2. a weak heart,
3. sinus or ear infections,
4. detachment of the retina,
5. bad posture when you stand normally, or if
6. you are overweight.

By far the greatest number of offenders are those in group five. You must be able to stand up completely straight and drop your shoulders down with ease. There should not be any trace of a stoop in your stance because the Headstand would, if anything, cement it into place, possibly causing damage to the neck. So, while there is no doubt that the Headstand is a wonderful way of getting a great amount of work done all in one posture, don't forget that this work can also be done by a combination of other postures which are very much easier.

It is really best to learn the Headstand with a teacher because it is almost impossible in the beginning to judge whether your head is at exactly the correct angle and whether you are in fact standing completely vertical in your upside-down position. It is surprisingly easy to develop a Leaning Tower of Pisa effect without even knowing that it is happening–until one morning you wake up and find your neck is jammed solid. So if you must learn the Headstand, be in no hurry about it, and if possible find a good teacher and, if you cannot find a teacher, then get someone, anyone, to tell you whether you are in fact standing absolutely vertically when you have completed the posture.

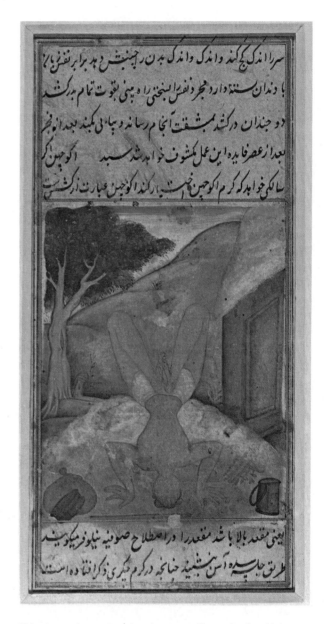

This sixteenth- or seventeenth-century illustration in a Yoga text translated into Persian clearly shows the unchanged tradition of the yogi's headstand, Sirshasana.

Strength in the neck is obviously one requirement in the Headstand. But, strangely enough, another of the keys to learning it successfully is flexibility at the lower end of the spine. Without this flexibility it is far more difficult to rise upside down in a slow

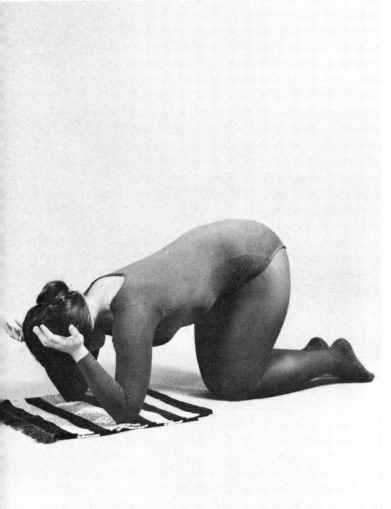

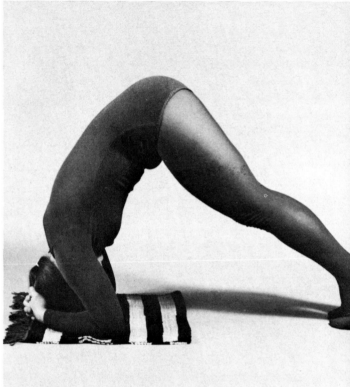

and controlled movement and to adjust once you are in position.

It would require a book to detail every single benefit that can be obtained from the Headstand. First the spine itself is helped to achieve a good balance and a correct position. The load is taken off the lower part of the spine, which in the normal course of events carries the greatest weight and is subject to the biggest strains. The circulation to the lungs and the brain is vastly improved, and the veins in the legs are relieved of pressure. The whole of the abdominal region is decongested and any displacement of the inner organs tends to be corrected. Venous blood is drained away and automatically replaced by fresh arterial blood – the basis of a renewed health and youth. The quality of this blood is improved by the fact that when the body is upside down the weight of the intestines rests on the diaphragm, which in turn presses on the lungs, so that they are usually emptied much better. This enhanced blood also finds its way in extra amounts to the brain. If the Headstand is learned during youth, then the capillaries of the brain tend to develop the ability to accommodate the extra blood and there can be a large gain in mental effectiveness. If this asana is not learned until later, then an improvement will still take place but to a lesser extent owing to the fact that the capillaries will not be so well adapted for the purpose. Equally obviously, if the blood pressure is too high or the capillaries stiff with sclerosis, then the extra blood can cause damage to the miniature blood vessels. Although detachment of the retina can be adversely affected by the Headstand, astigmatism, shortsight, etc. can only benefit from the extra flush of blood.

How to do this wonder posture? There are many versions and methods and some teachers are adamant that their particular way is best. The following method is a quite generally recognized way to the pose.

Kneel down. Form a cup with your clasped hands on the ground in front of you. Your elbows should be at shoulder width and the upper part of your arms should run straight down to the ground from your shoulders. Into the cup formed by your hands you fit the head so that the crown of the head is on the ground in between your hands.

Now the secret of learning the Headstand easily lies in *not* attempting to stand straight upright in the beginning. Simply straighten your knees and then inch your feet in towards your head very gently until you begin to find yourself balancing on your head. Do not attempt to lift your legs up but content yourself with balancing with your legs just a

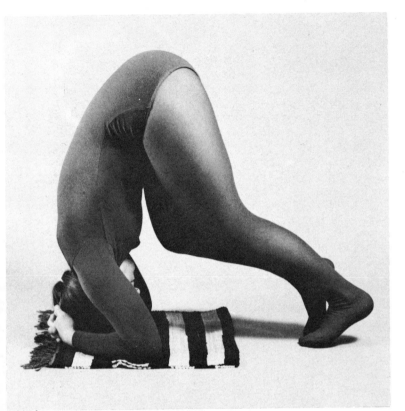
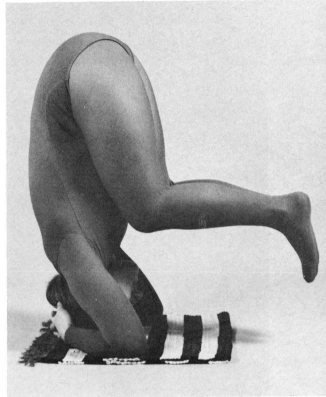

The first four steps of the Headstand. Until you can balance comfortably as above, do not try to straighten up.

couple of inches off the floor. Only when you can do this really easily should you try to lift your legs up. And then *never* try to push off to the upright position one leg at a time. Always raise *both* legs very slowly up *together*. If you feel yourself over-balancing, then either lower yourself down again or collapse into a ball and roll over. Now if you follow this rule, it is almost impossible to hurt yourself by falling over. If, on the other hand, you insist on trying to hold an imperfect balance with your legs up, then the quite inevitable result is that you will fall over with a slow, heavy crash, like a tree to the call of 'Timber!'. It will also hurt. Learning the Headstand is remarkably good for cutting the ego down to size.

There is an alternative way to do the Headstand which some people find very much easier in the beginning because it gives a broader base for them to balance on. In this version you start as before by kneeling and forming a triangle with your clasped hands so that the elbows are directly below your shoulders. But this time you note the position of your elbows, unclasp your hands and put the hands where the elbows were. This gives you a three-point base, formed by your head and your two hands, on which to balance (see page 91).

Once again inch the feet in as far as you can. Now

bend one knee and place it on the elbow at the same side. Then put the other knee on the other elbow and you will be standing on your head in a bent-over position. Do this until you are completely confident. Then very slowly straighten both legs simultaneously and raise them into a vertical position.

It is tremendously important that no matter which method you use, your body should be in a straight line, and this can only be done if your head is in the correct position. Most people tend to put their forehead instead of their crown to the floor, thus producing a kink in the neck. You can tell when you are in a perfectly straight line because your muscles will be able to relax all up and down your body. You will in fact be performing a head balance—and the operative word is 'balance'. Do not try to point your toes. Concentrate on total relaxation and balance.

The length of time you remain upside down is up to you, but better come down too soon than stay up too long. A minute is plenty to begin with. Rely on your body telling you. If you feel at all uncomfortable, come down. If you find it hard to

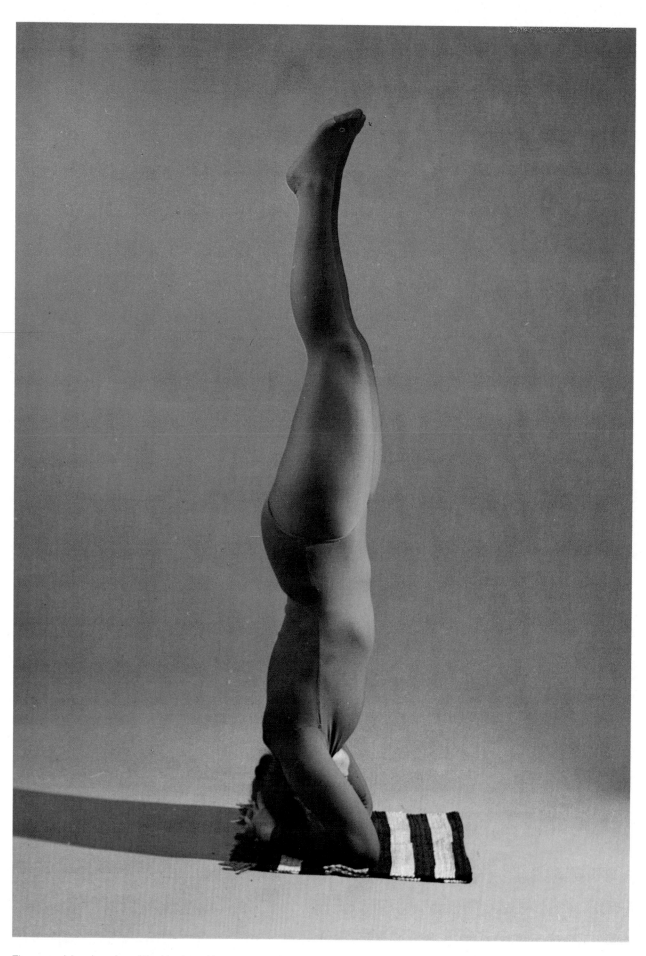

The cupped-hand version of the Headstand is more generally popular.

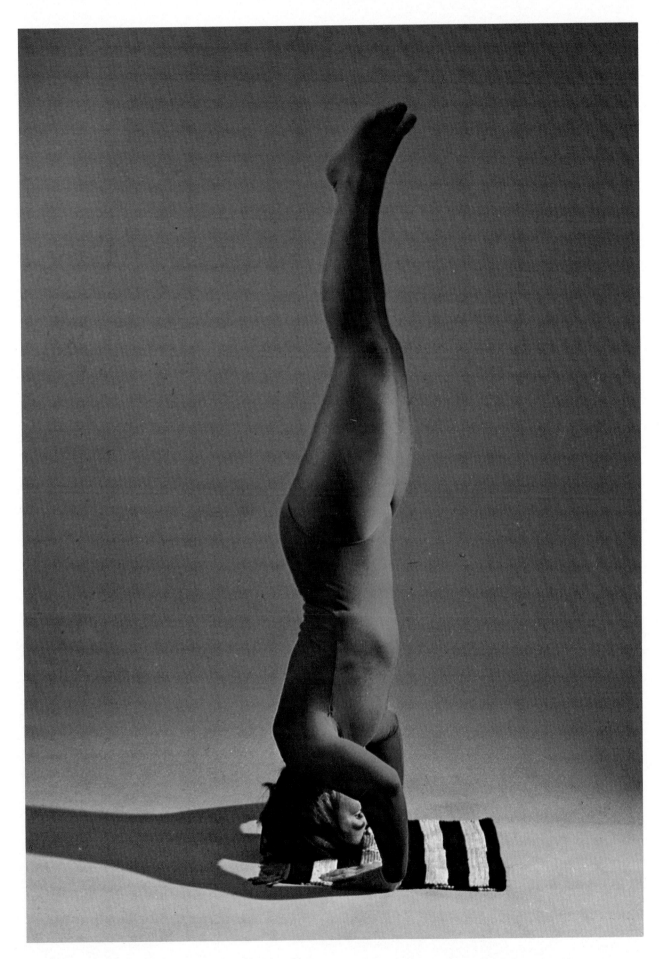

Another completed Headstand. Note the altered hand position.

breathe when upside down, the chances are that you are not properly balanced and that muscular tension is not allowing you to breathe easily. You should, by the way, be breathing through the nose.

Turning the whole body upside down is a fairly drastic form of exercise so do not try to get up immediately after you have been attempting the Headstand. Remain in a kneeling position with your head down and touching your clasped hands, and only very slowly straighten up from this position after a rest of about half a minute.

No Yoga posture should be practised in isolation from the whole system and the Headstand is no exception, in spite of its remarkable number of virtues. B.K.S. Iyengar reports that people who use the Headstand without its counter pose tend to become aggressive and quick-tempered. If the Headstand is the king of asanas, then the Shoulder Stand is its queen and practice of the Headstand should always be followed by practice of the Shoulder Stand.

It is not advisable to try working exactly to a timetable and a clock in the upside-down posture. Maybe the time spent upside down is being increased by only ten seconds per day, but even this may become too much for someone. Therefore rely, as you should always do, on listening to the language of your body.

In any upside-down posture there are two sensations of a rise in pressure. The first comes in a matter of a few seconds and will fade as the body adjusts to the upside-down position. The second rise is the warning for you to come down. When you begin, it may take place almost immediately on top of the first rise so that you will be warned that you have had enough in as short a time as fifteen seconds. If you are younger, fitter, more relaxed, it will be delayed, and you may not feel the rise for many minutes. But take no chances at all. The moment you feel a suspicion of a rise for the second time, come down. There is absolutely no virtue in remaining upside-down for the sake of it. It does no good, only damage.

If you feel uncomfortable in any upside-down pose at any time, the chances are that you are not performing it correctly and are building in tensions. Find an expert to check your technique, and, if you still feel wrong, well – did you check your blood pressure before starting?

Alternative bases from which to begin the Headstand: the cupped-hand version *(left)* and the triangular version *(right)*.

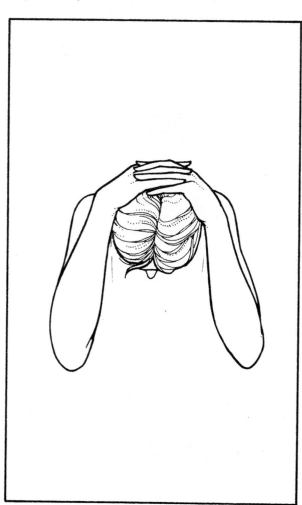

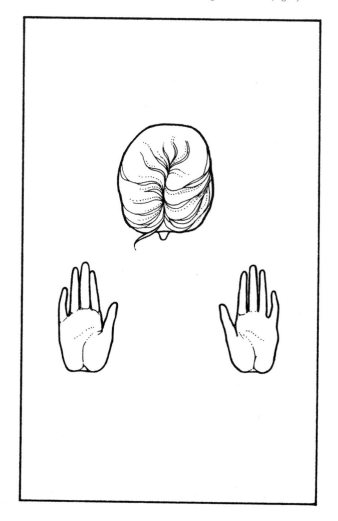

STILLNESS AND RELAXATION– THE DIFFERENCE

Yoga is, if nothing else, the art of total and perfect relaxation. Let us see what tension is and why it drains so much energy from us.

Take a simple physical illustration: two teams in a tug of war. The piece of rope is not heavy. A small child could pull it along with one hand. For argument's sake let us say it needs 10 pounds of energy to move the rope. Now suppose that you attach one end of the rope to a man who can pull a weight of 100 pounds. To pull the rope away from that man you need to be able to pull 10 pounds for the rope plus 100 for the man: a total of 110 pounds. Suppose we even things up and have another man on the other end, also pulling 100 pounds of weight, what happens? A small child with a 10-pound pull can draw the rope one way or the other. We can add two more men at each end and, so long as each of them pulls the same 100 pounds, the child will still be able to move the rope with a 10-pound pull. But look what we have: it now takes a total of 310 pounds to move the rope, and, worse still, the total amount of energy involved is 610 pounds, 300 pounds a side plus the odd 10 needed to move the rope!

This is what tension means to you – 610 pounds of energy used up to do a 10-pound job. Take a tiny tension in your body and then multiply it by the number of individual muscles or muscle fibres; the total energy drain is simply enormous. Each worry is an energy drain. If you are worrying at the same time as you are going your work, you have to summon up enough energy not only to cope with the worry but also to cancel it out.

Of course, there is nothing wrong with a certain amount of stress. We were built to cope with it and in fact it stimulates. Come to that, if we do not have enough stress in our lives we often go out and create it for ourselves. Sometimes we do it by proxy, going to watch a thrilling movie or a football match, but sometimes we do it more directly. The well-to-do young playboy who does not have a financial worry in the world may take up motor racing or become an amateur steeplechase jockey, risking his neck for a prize which means nothing in comparison to his personal fortune. Of course this need for stress is a symptom of an aimlessness in life that Yoga can conquer, but it does also show that stress is not an uncontrollable bogey. Properly controlled, it is positively healthy.

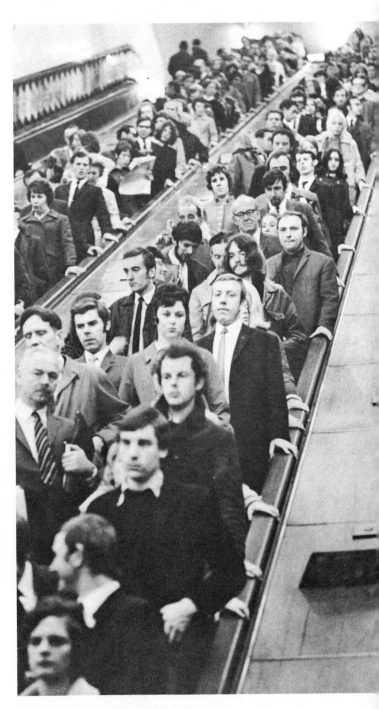

The 'rush hour'. Can you rush home to relaxation?

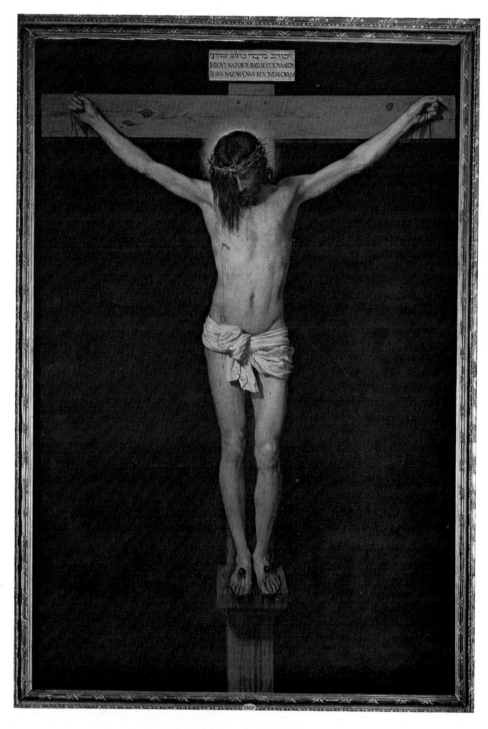

Probably no other religion has ever become so distorted as Christianity. Once the fatal flaw of sex repression was introduced, this doctrine of universal love changed its symbol from that of a fish to that of death by torture. Subsequently whole centuries of Christian art were tainted with violence. Most of its images reflect a mass of externally or internally disintegrated human beings, the natural consequence of attempting to deny parts of human existence. In the Orient, religions maintained a greater interest in personal integration with the result that the images of its gods and people are benign, and the faces which look down from temple walls are mostly peaceful, if not actually smiling. Compare 'The Crucified Christ' by Velasquez *(left)* with a seventeenth-century Tibetan bronze of Manjuri, the Buddhist god of wisdom *(opposite)*.

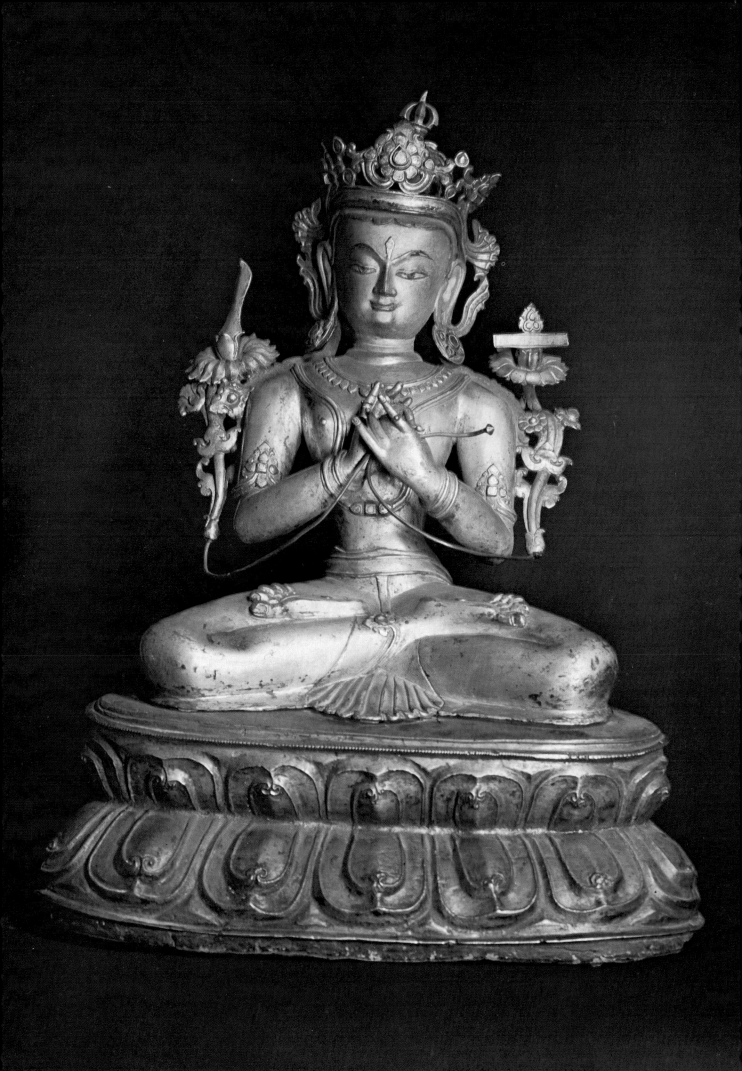

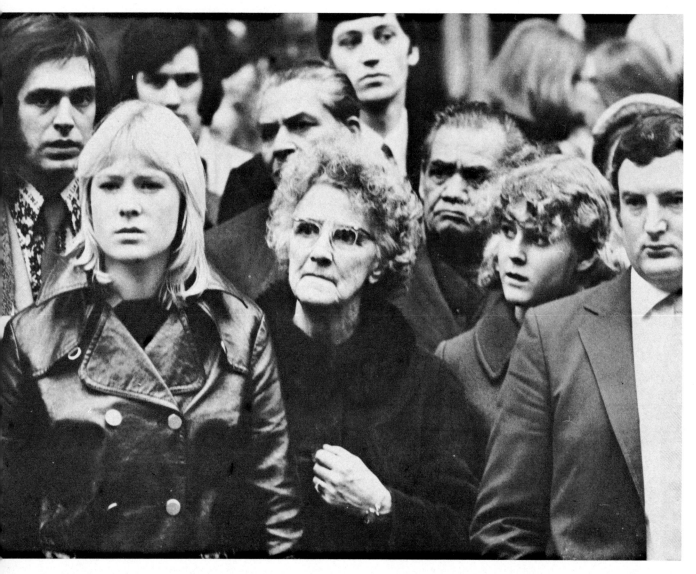

Faces in a big city street. There are getting to be so many people that man's only environment is man. A forest is only as green as the individual leaves. The quality of life is the quality of the people living it.

You may wonder how Yoga—coming from the far-away mountains of India and Tibet, where there is no traffic, no rush and bustle of crowded streets—has become so closely concerned with the elimination of nervous tension? The yogis know that you need peace of mind in order to ascend to superconscious awareness. Until the body and the mind have been brought under complete control, this state of consciousness cannot be achieved. The classic texts use the simile that you can only see the bottom of a pool when the surface water is calm.

Anybody can learn the first and most important posture which leads to total relaxation. It is at the same time both the simplest and yet the most difficult to do correctly. Superficially, all you do in the **Savasana** or **Corpse Pose** is just lie flat on your back on the floor stretched out and making no more movement than a corpse—but with one exception, you are breathing. However, to do the pose successfully you must recognize the vital difference between relaxation and stillness. Stillness can sometimes be forced onto a body but relaxation never can be. To examine the difference more closely let us return to the tug-of-war metaphor. If you take a piece of string, wind it round your hands, pull it tight and rest your hands on the table, the string will be completely still but it will not be relaxed. It will also be using up your energy as you hold it tight. Unwind it from your hands and let it lie on the table in front of you. It is equally still but now it is relaxed. The only strength needed to move it is that

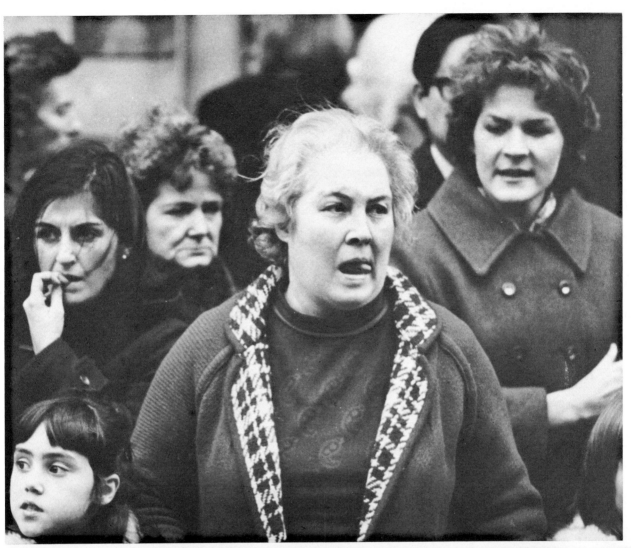

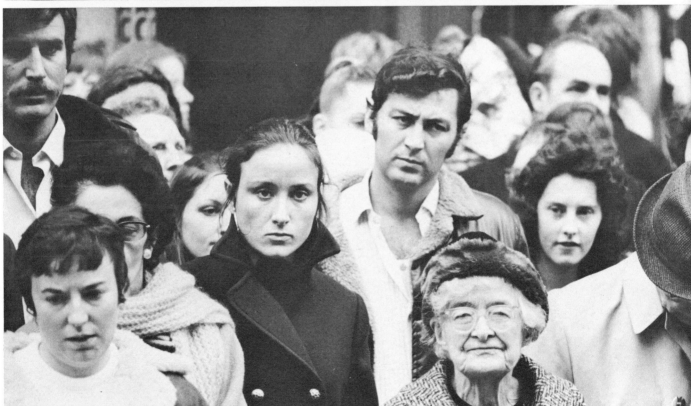

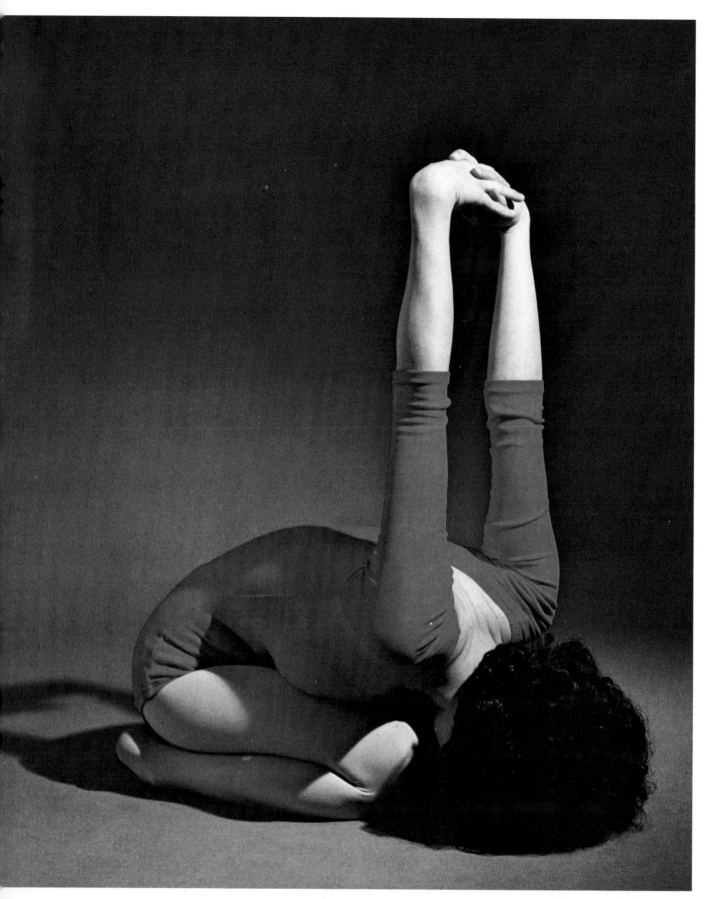

Above: Bowing forward until the head touches the ground is the almost universal symbol of humility; it is virtually impossible to remain in such a posture and retain a feeling of arrogance. This is another Yoga Mudra (see page 79). Its stretching action helps to awaken the psychic centres.

Opposite: Almost all Oriental religions have absorbed some of the techniques of Yoga. Their paintings consequently incorporate mandala designs, which form visual reminders of the order of the cosmos.

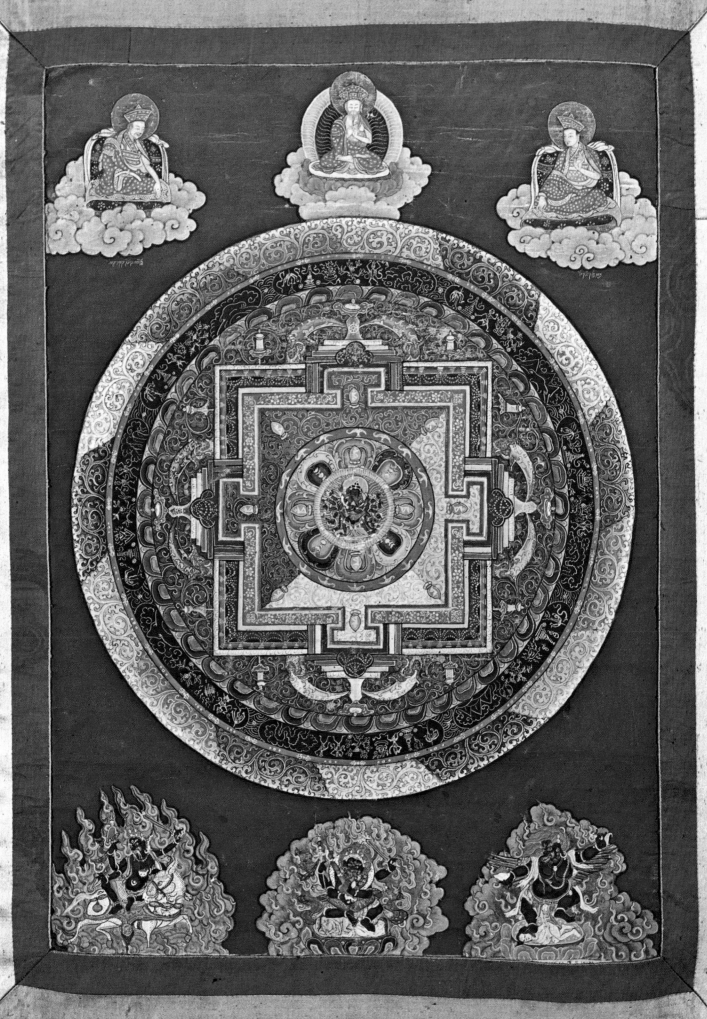

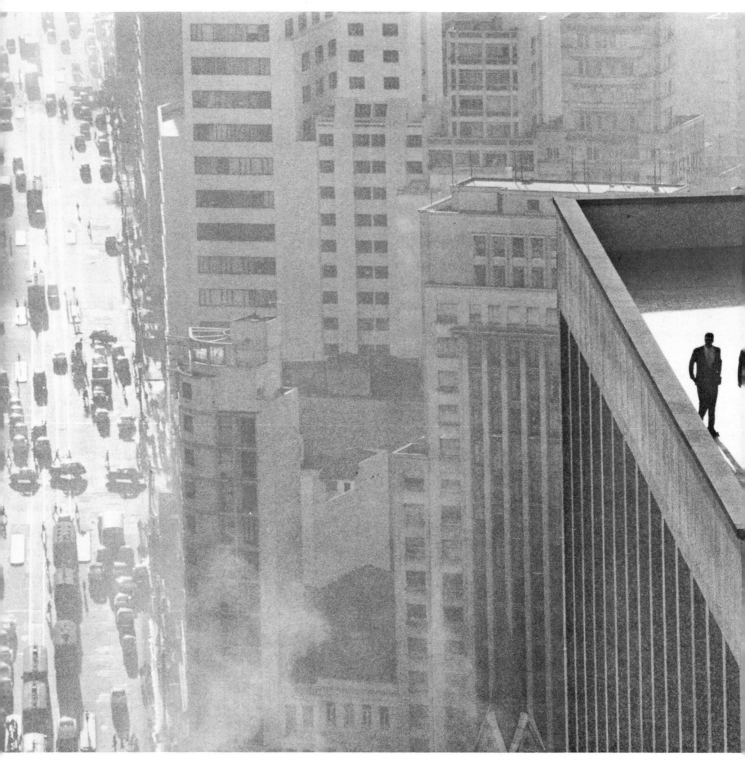

The concrete jungle of Sao Paulo, Brazil, and the industrial pollution of Dusseldorf, West Germany. Even though man is capable of creating his own environment, there is a limit to the amount of change which can be made if human life is to be maintained. Have we reached that limit?

of a fingertip. Add to this relaxed condition the notion that the string is alive and has a beating pulse inside it and you get some idea of the condition your body will be in when it is relaxed.

Forcing stillness onto your body, from the outside so to speak, is not relaxation. Relaxation comes when there is stillness inside you. You can achieve it by divesting yourself of your hang-ups one by one, and when a hang-up goes it may just dissolve or it may go out with a bang so that you shake or even cry. You may well find that you are a very lively corpse indeed. It is very important to grasp this point. The aim of the Corpse Pose is *not* to lie still.

The aim is to *relax*. Eventually through the relaxation will come the stillness.

Savasana is best practised on a firm foundation and not; but definitely *not*, on a springy bed. At the most all you need is very thin foam or a doubled blanket beneath you. The surface you use should be completely flat so that you are not lying uphill or

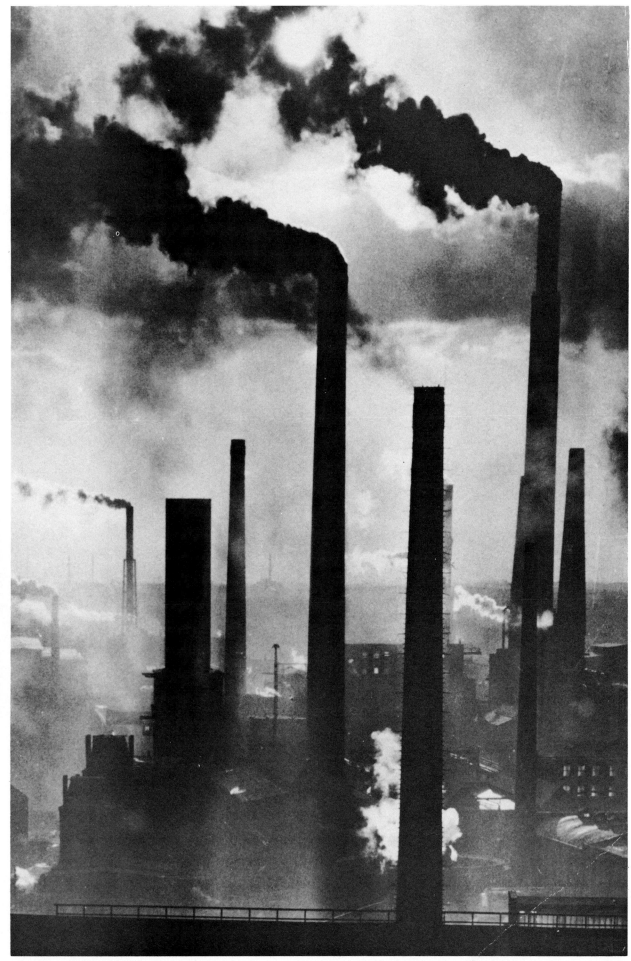

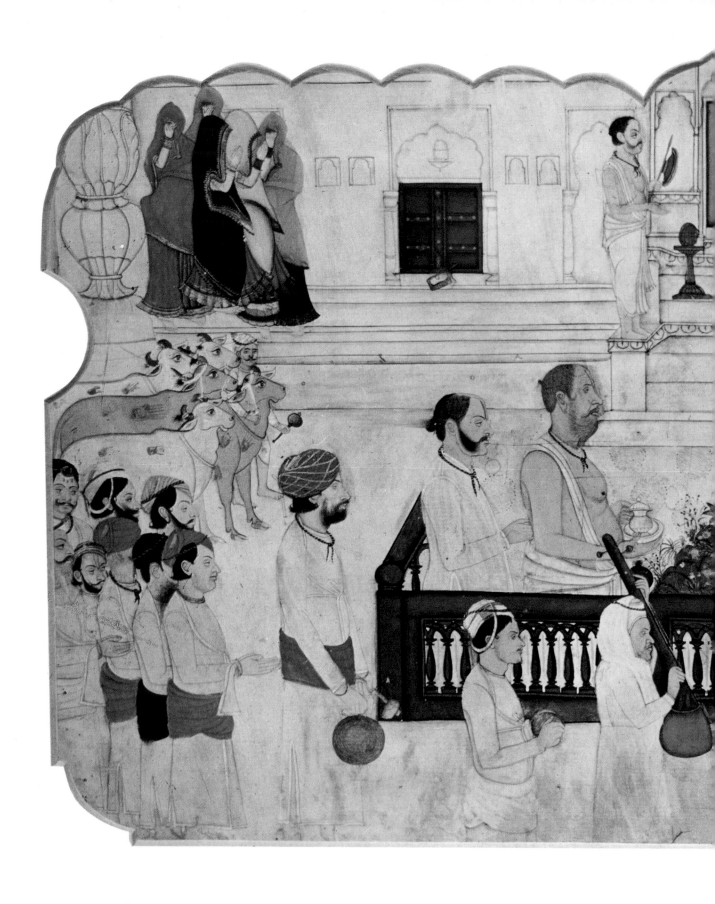

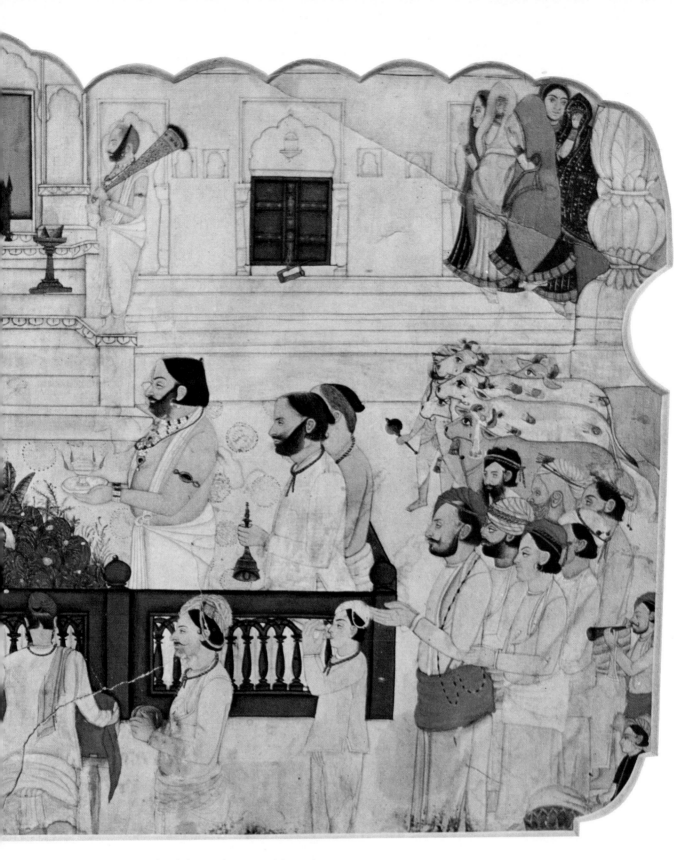

Yoga is not a religion since it has no dogmas and demands
no beliefs. Bhakti Yoga, the Yoga of devotion, is the nearest
Yoga comes to religion. It is considered by some to be the
easiest of Yogas since it demands no long training or
discipline; all it asks is that the follower should turn his love
to the divine. This early nineteenth-century Indian painting
shows worshippers at a shrine sacred to Krishna.

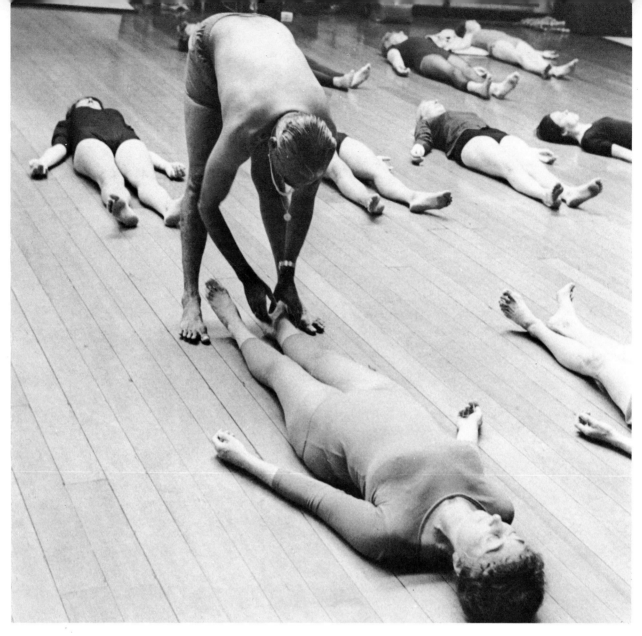

In Savasana, the Corpse Pose, the limbs must be positioned exactly symmetrically.

downhill. The room should preferably be warm enough for you to lie without a covering, but if it is at all draughty or cold then you can use a light blanket or rug to keep you warm. This is quite important because when your body is cold the muscles automatically tense in order to create heat for you.

The pose begins with the accurate and comfortable placing of the body on the floor. Sit in the centre of the rug with your knees drawn up and in your mind learn to recognize what is called the 'median line' of your body. This is a line which runs through the exact centre of your body from your feet to the very tip of your head. Stretch out one leg and then the other so that your feet are a few inches apart and each leg is the same distance from the median line. Now lean back onto your elbows and look down your body to make sure that you are still in a dead straight line, easing your buttocks off the floor and adjusting them for comfort and straightness. Lie back and again wriggle your buttocks comfortable and squint down your body to check the alignment. Place your arms on the floor with the hands about five inches from your sides, palms up.

At this point you may find that your spine is stretching and so you should raise yourself up and flatten it one vertebra at a time until you are lying with your spine in a dead straight line and with as much of it touching the floor as possible. Finally lower your head to the ground so that the line of the jaw is roughly vertical to the ground. On the first occasion that you try this pose, it is good to have someone to help you to line up. Most of us have developed lopsided tensions and it is quite an exception to find someone who does not at first lie with the head tilted slightly to one side.

Why all this fuss about lying so completely straight and flat? The reason is that the tilt toward the stronger side of the body creates a drain of energy from the lower side to the ground. When the two halves of the body on either side of the median line are completely balanced, then so are the energy circuits in the body and the energy remains "locked" inside it. Consequently a recovery of general vitality is much quicker than if there is a pranic "leak" on one side.

Assuming that you have arranged yourself in a balanced position, you now begin the process of conscious relaxation. If your body is truly straight and not at all twisted, you may straightaway begin to feel a certain lightness but for a beginner this is not likely and so you must start working at relaxing. The simplest way is to begin at the feet and work upwards.

Transfer your mind to your left foot; relax. Then to your right foot; relax it. Your left knee; relax it. Your right knee; relax it. Your thighs. Now move to your hands and work your way up your arms. Then work up your body and finally, and most important, relax your face: your throat, your mouth, your nose, your tongue, and your eyes.

Now concentrate on your breathing. It should slow down gradually, and the outward breath should take slightly longer than the inward breath. For many people who are worn out and badly in need of sleep this period of quiet breathing will be enough to send them off. Sleep is not the aim of Savasana but, if you need sleep that badly, then you should make the most of it. Incidentally, the sleep which comes *after* you have had a preliminary relaxation is of a much better quality than that which comes when you drop off with your mind bubbling from the unquiet memories of the day. Still, Yoga relaxation is conscious relaxation, and at some point you must begin *not* to fall asleep but to continue on a definite process of relaxation.

It is very unlikely that you will achieve a total relaxation immediately. If you can have someone who is skilled to check your degree of relaxation, this can help you along quickly but you can still manage by yourself. All you need to do is repeat the check from your feet to your head, relaxing your muscles consciously. At this point some odd things may happen to you, especially if you are really wound up about life. You may begin quite literally to unwind, and the result is not unlike a spring breaking loose. You may find that your body twitches. Your breathing may become irregular. When you try to control it, you may giggle or even burst into tears. Whatever happens, just let it happen, only every time bring your mind back to slow, gentle breathing–after you have had your laugh or cry. Every time you have a break-out of emotion you will find that your body is lying straighter and flatter on the floor.

When and if you are reasonably calm, you can begin recharging yourself. As you lie on the ground, think of your body energy current flowing up your back, over the top of the head, and down the front of the body. The energy is stored at the manas cakra, which is in the region of the solar plexus. So as you lie on the ground visualize the energy flowing over you and into your solar plexus. Its downward movement from your head is made at the same time as you exhale. With this exhalation of breath, you also send out your ego so that you hand yourself back to the cosmos. You will feel not that you are lying on the earth but that the earth is pushing you up. Even the very first time you try this posture you may suddenly have a flash of revelation that your body is fixed to this planet

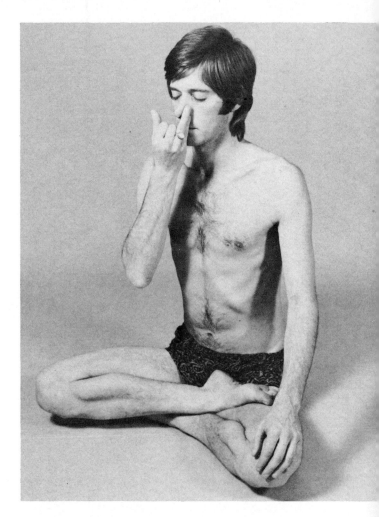

Nadi Shodana, a form of alternate nostril breathing. Breathe out and in through one nostril, while holding the other closed. Change over and breathe out and in through the other nostril. Change back and so on, maintaining a steady rhythm. Nadi Shodana is a tranquillizer and cleanser.

racing through space, an enormous space bigger than you have ever dreamed of. This may be your first glimpse of superconsciousness.

All the time you are lying down you will feel yourself getting longer and heavier so that it becomes a real effort to bring yourself back to everyday life. Because you may have gone so far out of yourself, you should allow a little time to come down to earth again. When your time is up, you deepen your breathing and quicken it. Then roll over onto your right side and bend your knees and arms so that they tend toward the foetal position. Lie in this position until you feel yourself to be integrated again. Then stretch. Roll over on the other side and stretch and then onto your back. Finally sit up and come back to the world. You will find yourself immensely refreshed. Half an hour of Savasana is worth a couple of hours of sleep.

In the beginning it will probably take you at least ten minutes to become even partly relaxed in Savasana and thirty minutes will be the shortest worthwhile session you can have. But as you become more practised, you will be able to reach deep relaxation in a few minutes so that even a ten-minute Savasana can be a real boost during the day.

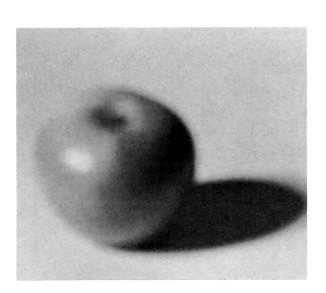

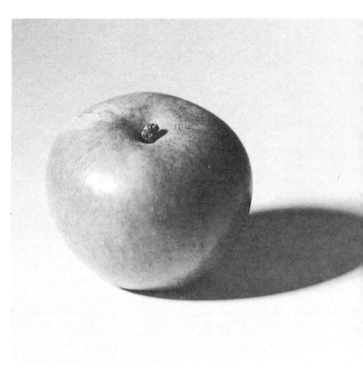

This page: In meditation the object which is viewed remains the same. The quality of the image depends on the observation and training of the viewer. Increased awareness inevitably brings an increase in the quality of life.

Opposite: In Yoga, the mental and the physical are balanced. Swami Yogeshwaranand is the respected head of Yoga Niketan, a small but selective ashram specializing in awareness techniques and long meditation. However, the Swamiji will quite happily lead young fit students in a Hatha Yoga session vigorous enough to leave them breathless—he is currently in his eighty-seventh year.

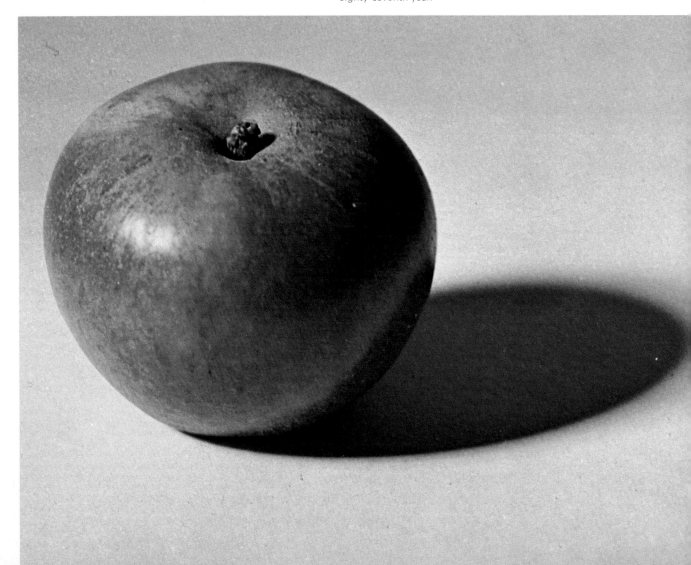

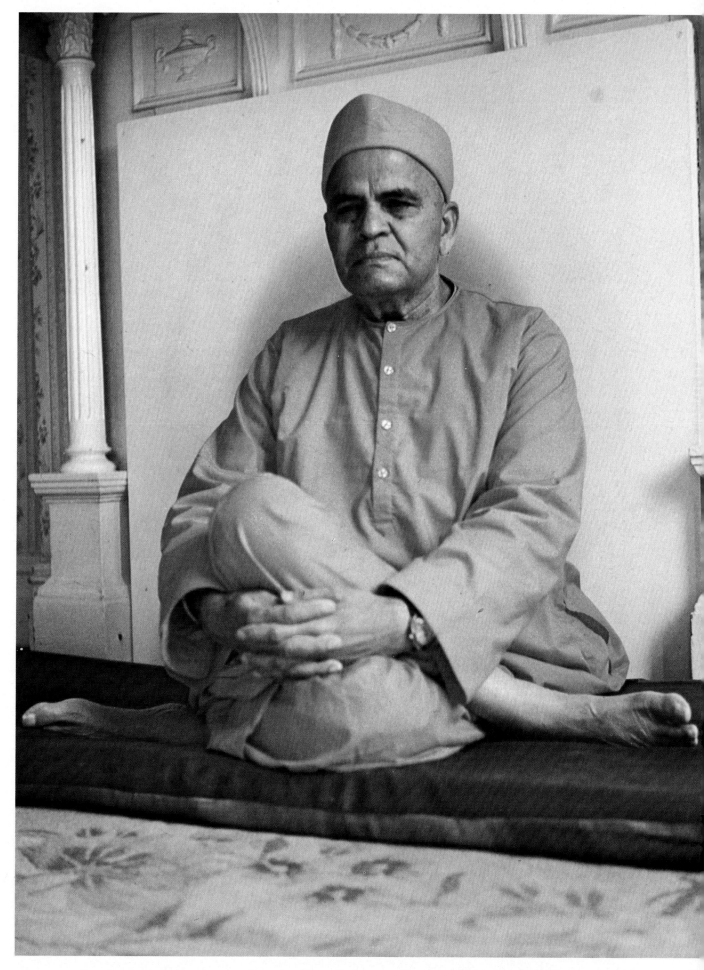

THE CENTRALLY-HEATED MIND

'Yoga is the control of the waves of the mind. Normally the self is identified with these waves, but it is possible to free it so that it rests on its own.'

Yoga sutras of Patanjali

Within the body of man and mammals is an automatic control which keeps the body working at its most effective temperature. The outside temperature may go up or down, the fingers may go cold, or the brow sweat from the heat, but the crucial inner organs in a human body maintain their own temperature.

The great aim of Yoga is to create a similar mental condition so that the mind remains unaffected by the many outside pressures that impinge upon it daily. Two things must be understood. Firstly, this does not mean that the mind is numbed, and secondly it is a condition which cannot be achieved by force. Forceful stilling of the mind is repression and both the yogis and Western psychologists have long since recognized the evil of this.

Western society is full of disciplines imposed from the outside. There are so many and they are imposed from such an early age in our childhood that it is often difficult for people even to recognize them. Guilt so buttresses our mental makeup that shame is commonplace. The removal of conditioned guilt is the first and most important step that any Western educated person can take on the path into Yoga. In some ways it is the process that is attempted in any psychotherapy.

Successful yogis are happy people. The discipline that comes from the inside is less a discipline and more an act of love. The discipline which says on a barrack square, 'Left turn! Right turn! Left turn! About turn! About turn!', is not really discipline. It is merely 'conditioning'. It only becomes a discipline if the recruit who is being drilled feels the need for this training.

The sum of peace in any community is the sum of the inner peace of each person living in it. The incredible importance of all this should not be hard to see. It means that the peace and survival of the whole planet depend on the quality of the *inner life of each human being living here*. A forest can only be as green as the individual leaves on each tree.

Think of the disruptive influence that some people have. If you examine the psyche of such

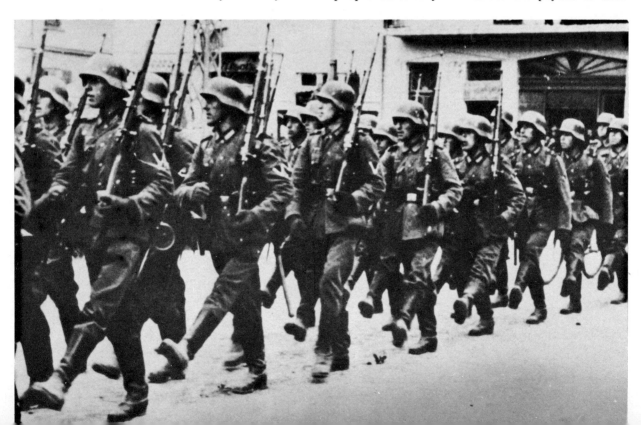

people, you will invariably find that there is a veritable tornado of unhappiness at work within the core of the personalities. And if just one madman with a rifle can turn the life of a whole community from happiness into terror, what then is the effect of even one man full of inner torment who has the power to order many men with rifles, be they mad or not.

Make a little experiment. Think right now of the things which are forced on you somehow. Who is the person or group of persons who is causing you to go through all this trouble? The chances are that you will not have to look far before you discover that it is somebody's self-interest that is responsible – someone's greed or possibly someone's wish for power over other people.

Think quickly. Do you have any greed or any wish for power over other people? Be honest. Well, never mind. You can come back to that one.

Reverse the process and think about those people who bring you happiness. Practically the first thing you will find out about them is that they do not try to dominate you and they do not always want things, either from you or from other people.

If you now think back to the various physical Yoga exercises that you have been doing, you will see that part of their purpose has been to create within you a condition of awareness. If you have been working on these Yoga postures with the right amount of concentration, you will have found out many things about your own body. Let us take an example. There is a yogic joke that the Shoulder Stand is the most successful slimming exercise in the system. It's a joke because there is very little effect on the muscle corset of the abdomen in this posture, but what does happen is that as you stand, upside down, your head is pointing straight at your stomach, and the longer you stand there the more aware you become that the stomach bulging just above you is much, much too large. You just cannot avoid seeing it. It's no good shutting your eyes either because you can feel the weight of that over-size waistline pressing down on your breathing system.

Yoga also has a whole range of other methods for developing the ability to become aware of yourself and the world. When the yogis talk about 'awareness' they are usually referring to the ultimate, 'transcendental' state of awareness, in which you cease to

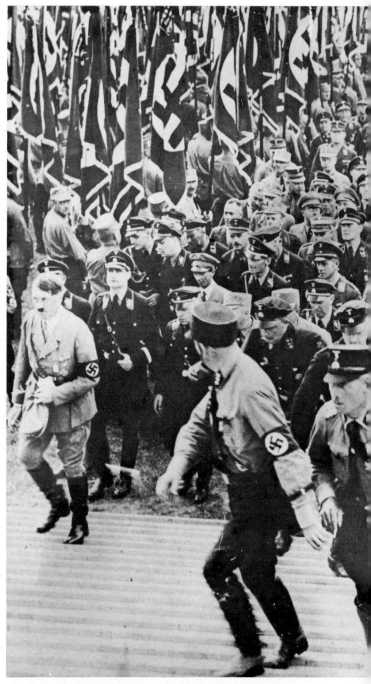

One man full of inner torment? Adolf Hitler: German occupation of France *(opposite)* and 1933 Nuremberg Rally *(above)*.

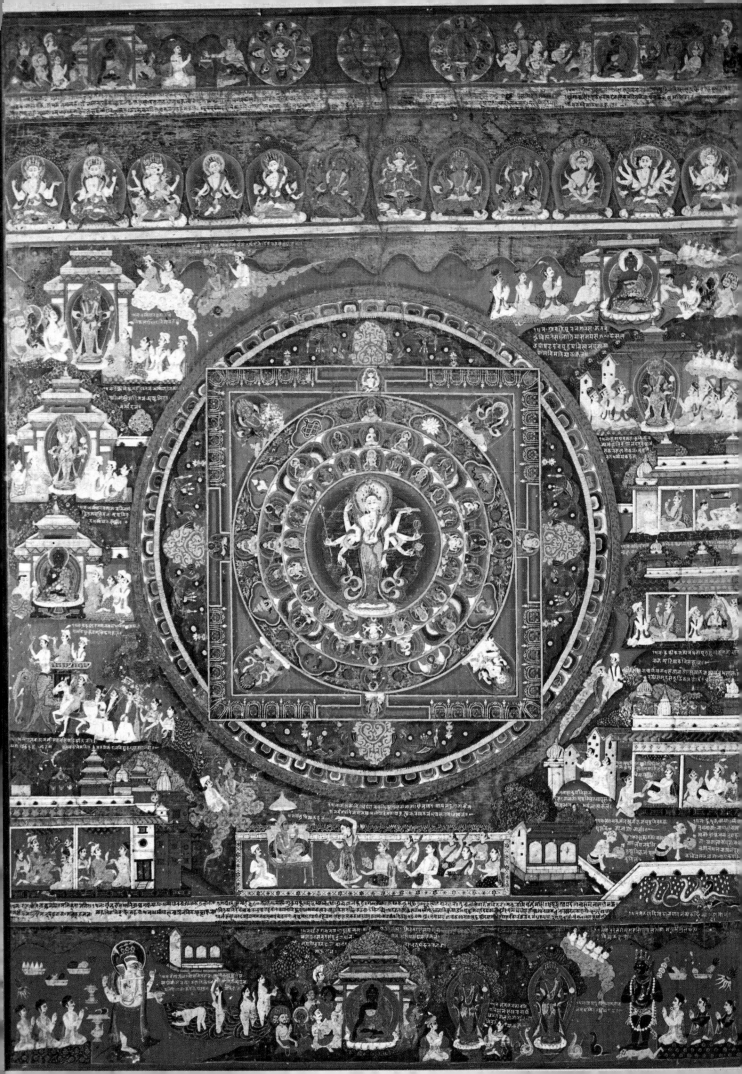

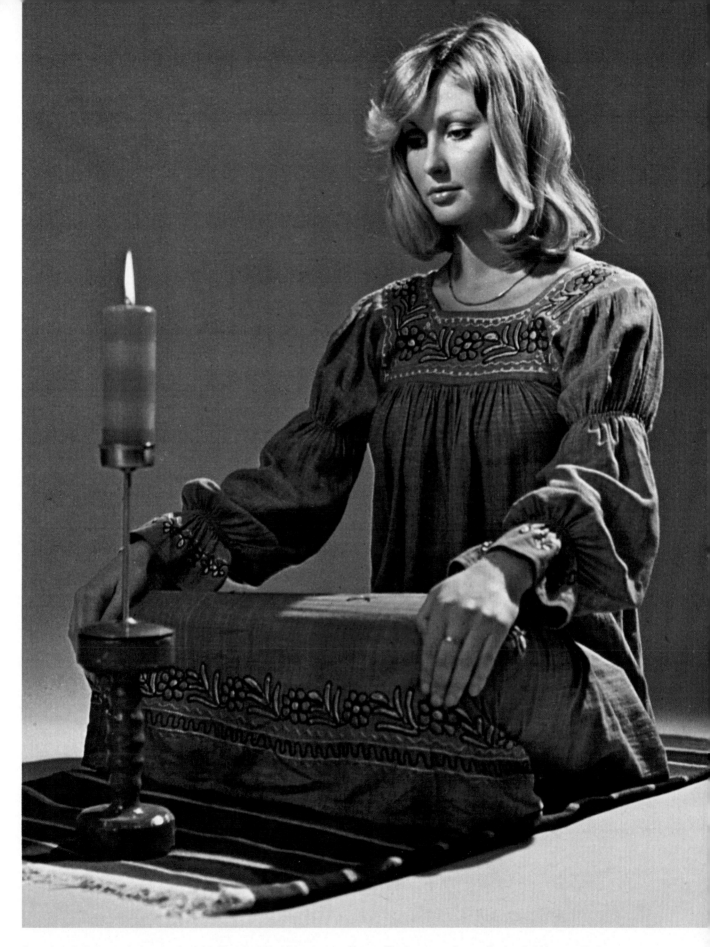

Opposite: Religious paintings such as this Nepalese Buddhist tanka could be used either as an object for meditation or alternatively as a visual religious history for a non-literate community.

Above: The least complex meditational aid is a candle flame, to which 'tratakam', an unblinking gaze, is applied.

be bound by time, space, and the body. Some people can slip in and out of this state quite easily and, if you can remember far enough back into your own childhood, you may even realize that you had this ability at times. However, before reaching transcendental awareness there are other degrees of awareness which, while providing stepping stones to the transcendental state, are of immense value for daily living.

How, then, to reach conditions of awareness? The problem lies not in the difficulty of the route but in its quite extraordinary simplicity. Neither the route nor the goal may turn out to be anything like what you expected. In fact, you may not realize that you are travelling at all–until you find you have arrived.

The key to the whole system of Yoga meditation and the yogic way of life is to learn how to examine everything objectively–especially yourself. Part of the trick is to recognize right from the start that you view the world through the spectacles of your own experience and life-style. In other words, you have to recognize what sort of a trip you are on before you can decide if it is right for you. Do not try to ignore or dismiss personal preferences. What do you gain from your particular way of living? Are you on a success jag? Or an ego trip? Or perhaps a "self-punishment" trip, in which you unconsciously cheat yourself of happiness? The importance of recognizing your trip is obvious yet some people manage to go apparently a long way into the yogic life without doing so.

Yoga supplies a number of mental exercises which help you to think about your own thought processes. During our schooling we are usually doing no more than feeding facts into the "computing" area of our brains. Visualizing is something that is usually severely frowned upon by the school-fact crammers. It is called "daydreaming" and often heavily punished, with the result that children who are schooled out of dreaming tend to become zombies, controlled by whatever outside influence happens to affect their "computer" brains, which is very convenient for politicians. Involuntary day-dreaming is certainly not desirable but a controlled voluntary daydreaming is a path to full mental control and self-realization. You must learn to separate external influences and internal influences and to explore the possibilities of yourself.

Many of the Yoga techniques require that you close your eyes and make your mind go to work– recalling images at will from your memory and constructing from them. In fact, this is what is done by most writers and artists, who are visualizers. Now *you* must learn how to see pictures in your own mind.

Firstly, lie down comfortably. Close your eyes. Now relax but try not to go to sleep.

Allow images to come and go in your mind, no matter what they are.

When you feel settled, keep your eyes closed and turn them upward and a little inwards with the thought: 'I am going to look into my brain. I am going to place there only those things that I want to place there.'

You are going to make notes and so you will need something to write on "inside your brain". Choose whatever you like. Say to your brain: 'I want a plain writing pad (or a blackboard or a slate or whatever).'

Conjure up inside your brain a picture of the item, with a clean space on which to write.

Now order yourself a pencil and a rubber, or a chalk and some cloth, not a pen and ink, because you will want to rub things out at times.

Give yourself a simple order. Write the numbers from one to ten. See your hand actually doing the writing. Put a dash in between each number like this:

$$1 - 2 - 3 - 4 - 5 - 6 - 7 - 8 - 9 - 10$$

Now rub it all out. This time you write the whole of the alphabet in the same way:

$$A - B - C - D - E - F - G - H - I - J \text{ and so on.}$$

When you have done this, you again erase what you have written in your mind. Next you begin on the numbers again and you write this time from 1 to 100. But you write in different colours, changing the colour at the end of each group of twenty. Say up to 20 is in green; up to 40 is then in orange; 40 to 60 is in yellow; 60 to 80 in blue, and 80 to 100 in red.

By this time you are likely to feel quite tired so you write out in front of you the words 'I am not going to sleep'–and then you relax and have a rest. Open your eyes if you wish.

When you are ready, start again but with something slightly different.

Close your eyes.

In your mind, draw a series of vertical lines.

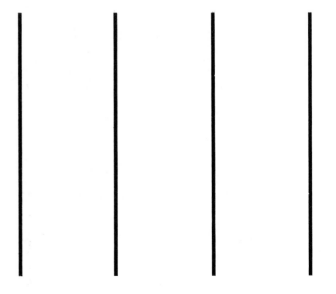

Wipe them off and now draw a series of horizontal lines.

Put the vertical lines back over them so that you have a grill.

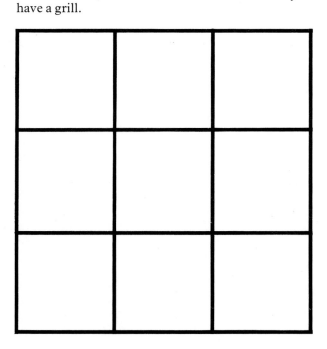

Wipe this off and draw a triangle.

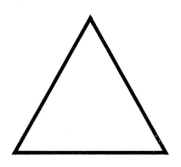

Now on top of it draw another triangle, upside down.

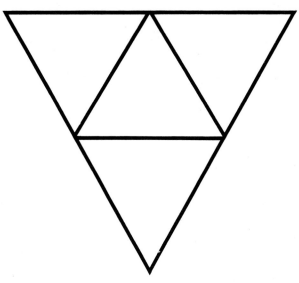

Place a dot in the very centre where the two triangles overlap.

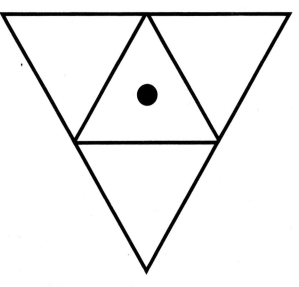

Think about the dot. Now relax and open your eyes. In your mind you have drawn a 'yantra', an aid to meditation which helps concentration. Overlapping triangles are very familiar in Yoga and are often used to symbolize aspects of infinity.

The mental exercises that you have just done are little more than mental push-ups, and they are probably just as dull to do, which is why they are often tiring. But to the enormous majority of people who have not been trained to visualize they can be extremely helpful in learning how consciously to put your mind to work – or to rest.

YOU ARE HERE AND NOW-SO LOOK

If you were to follow the path of creating only internal images, you might progress in fantasy but not in reality. You now know that your mind can work on its own and create an image where there is no physical counterpart. But you are dwelling inside a physical frame which has some pretty strict limitations, and now is the time to have a closer look at it. Bear in mind that examining your surroundings is not going to affect them, but it will make you more conscious of them and of yourself.

Take yourself out to a park or any place where you can watch toddlers playing and babies crawling. See how the youngsters look so intensely at any new thing that they encounter. Into the minds of children pour vast amounts of unrelated information, which the brain eventually begins to organize and to form into thought complexes. These complexes are then used for living. Not very surprisingly some of them develop no further. For example, if cornflakes come up for breakfast in the same old bowl with a plain plastic spoon day in day out, the child takes a quick glance and says to itself, 'Nothing new here. Same old plate, same old spoon, same old cornflakes. Just stuff the grub inside.' Hardly surprising that the plate is emptied in a flash and junior is asking to get down from table and away to other and more stimulating occupations. The 'breakfast' complex has been created.

This process of using thought complexes instead of original thought and observation can continue all the way through life so that people move about without actually thinking or even seeing what it is that is really going on around them. Consequently until they are hit by a gigantic disaster they may not notice how much things have been changing around them.

When you were a child, you needed to be able to use these condensed complexes in order to speed up on learning, but there comes a time in everyone's life when these thought complexes have to be looked at afresh. To take an example: just pick any word out of the blue. You will find that attached to this word are various ideas that go to make up your personal thought complex about it. Actually, those ideas which appear are likely to be only a part of the notions that make up the thought complex because those notions we find unpleasant tend to be kept hidden, although their effect on our lives may be even stronger than those we remember.

Go home to some room where you can be alone and quiet and where you feel safe. This matter of feeling safe is more important than may first appear: when you learn to look at yourself anew and where you are, you may find that it is not just a surprise to you but something of a shock.

Try to be sure that for a little while you will not be disturbed. Take the phone off the hook and lock the door. You are going to open your mind for the first time in maybe a very long while and an open mind is a sensitive one. You make of your room your own retreat or 'ashram'.

When you go into your little retreat, you should take something familiar and natural with you. The yogis of India often used a lotus blossom, the early Western mystics a rose. In Western cities neither roses nor lotus blossoms come easily to hand, but there are generally fruit and vegatables in the kitchen and these will do just as well, in fact possibly better. There is nothing high flown or rarified about looking at a lotus because the mental training can be done just as well with a bundle of alfalfa.

Going back to the children for a moment, you may have noticed how some of the young ones carry one particular doll around with them all the time. Sometimes it is not even a doll but just some old piece of rag which they will cling to at any cost—and usually somewhat to their mothers' embarrassment. These youngsters are dealing with the problem—and to them it poses an enormous threat—of things being 'I' and 'not I'. To a baby there is no difference between itself and the rest of the world. All belongs to baby and so all is baby. Learning that it is not all baby is a long and at times very painful and frustrating process. From the baby's point of view it is not taken out of its bed: the bed, a part of itself, is being removed. To retain its sense of being itself, and not something that can be dismembered at will by somebody else, a bit of the outer world is made into a portable 'I'—hence the dreadful old bit of rag which is carried around so closely all the time. It is a memory of the secure thought complexes when all the world was 'Me'.

In a way you are going to go back to this condition. So have you brought with you your familiar object? Say an apple or a potato? It is doubtless many a long year since you confused yourself with such an object so sit quietly and preferably cross legged and put it down in front of you. Now shut your eyes and

114

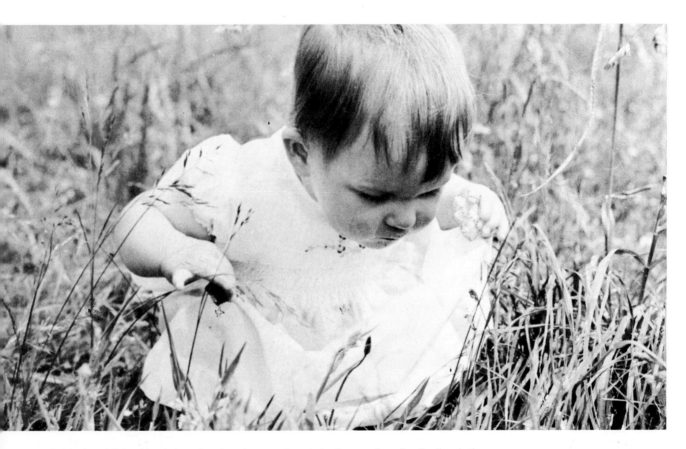

Babies are delighted by their explorations because there is for them no 'good' or 'bad', only the new.

quickly run through your superficial thought complex for the object, including trying to remember what various examples looked like. All right, so you know about potatoes or apples or whatever.

Now relax yourself as much as you can, open your eyes and look at the object you brought with you. Look at it as though you were seeing it for the first time. See how the light falls on it, and from which side. Is there enough light to cast a shadow? What is the colour of the shadow? What is the colour of the object itself? Do not answer too quickly. You may be drawing on the memory of an early thought complex. Hold the object in your hand and allow more information about it to flow in through your fingertips. Feel if it is rough or smooth, if it is heavy or light. Now put it down again.

Up to this point you have been looking *at* the object. Now you have some idea of *what* it is so you must next learn *where* it is. Say you have put it on a handkerchief: how far is it from the edges of the handkerchief? How far from the back? How far from the side? From the corners? How far away is the light? Where is the light in relation to the room—if you are in a room? If you are outside (and one day you must do this outdoors), where is the sun and how far away are the clouds?

Look down again at the object and ask yourself, 'How far away is the object from me?' You've come to the key question. You turn this previous question around and you ask, 'Where am *I* in relation to this object?'

Now you really begin. You examine yourself and your position in exactly the same way as you examined the position of the object. How far am I away from the light? How far am I from the walls? Am I central in this room? Does the light shine on

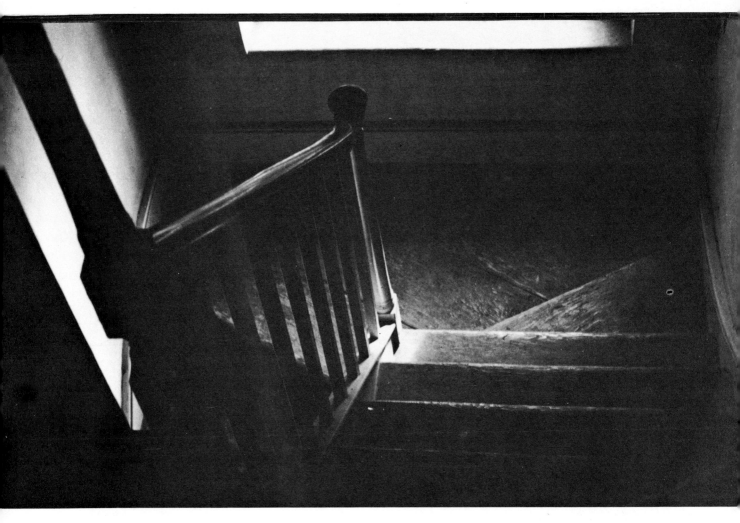

me? What is there here that is bigger than me? What is there that is smaller?

Try to think of yourself positioned in space. Do not look only at what is in front of you but turn round and find out what is behind you and what your relationship is to these things. Consider the fact that you are part of a living world, that you are surrounded by life. Say your name out loud and think of the earth whirling through space, a space which is filled with other worlds. Everything in this cosmos moves and everything within you moves.

Now quickly come back to earth. If you are not used to this sort of thing, you can scare the pants off yourself. This is why I suggested that you pick some place where you feel safe and happy. In your adult adventuring into the 'I' and the 'not I', you need your bit of reassurance, just as much as the child who clutches that favourite toy or bit of old rag. No need to be ashamed of it, you are after all only a very small portion of that enormous cosmos that we are all whirling about in.

The emotional releases that often take place in this sort of Yoga are sometimes of a tremendous and often unexpected intensity, but this is no reason to be frightened of them or worse still to attempt to dam them up. Tears are as much a natural release of tension as laughter or yawning. Keeping them back is the thing which sends psychiatrists happily into the yacht-owning income bracket. With the possible exception of attempting an overly quick release of the kundalini force, there is no experience in Yoga which you cannot either cry out or sleep off. If ever you do feel you are getting too upset, then you simply slow down a bit until you can make the next step with impunity.

If you have really concentrated during this session you will have acquired a new sense of dimension which will never leave you. And it need not be confined to periods of meditation. In fact, you should keep a constant check on yourself as you move around during the day.

As you walk along the road or go around a market, just quietly remind yourself that there is space all the way round you and then act as an observer of yourself. Mentally get out of yourself: move up and behind yourself. This enables you to look down and ask yourself the question, 'What's she up to now?' or 'he' if you happen to be a he. This simple sentence is not only a way of examining your physical actions, but a method of questioning the purpose of your activity. If you reply he/she is in a supermarket–remember, not 'I' but he or she– then you can examine why you are in a supermarket. Why and how has he/she arrived at this particular place at this particular time and could you or would you have been better off if you had gone elsewhere? Not just because the prices might be lower but because it might be part of a better life pattern for you. A continual examination of yourself for a period of time, say one week, may convince you of the need for considerable changes in the way you live your life.

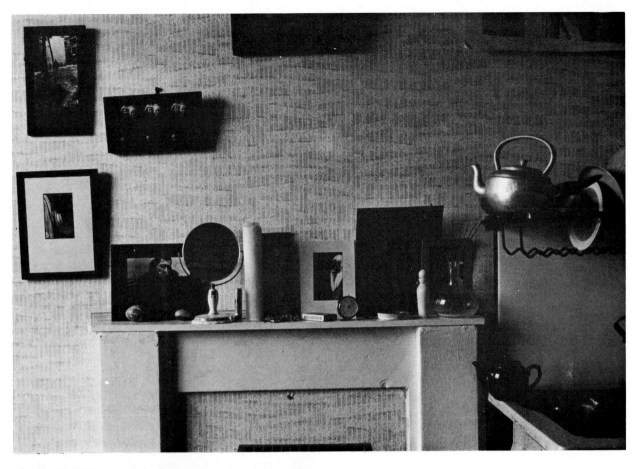

Go into any room in any house and look with the eye of an artist. Make no judgements—just see exactly what is there to be seen. Even your own home can look new to you.

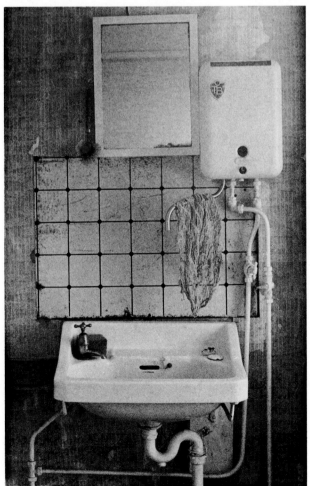

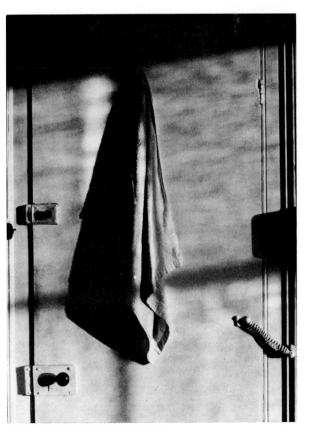

A SCREEN OF LOVE FOR JUST SITTING IN

'Sometimes I sits and thinks, and sometimes I just sits.'

An old country saying

The Zen Buddhists have a special word for just sitting; they call it 'zazen'. Some claim that it is the simplest and most direct form of meditation that you can use. All you need to do is sit comfortably, breathe very slowly and concentrate wholly on the feeling of the breath gently flowing in and out of your nostrils. You may find that this will bring considerable peace right away, but on the other hand you may find that all you get is the churning of your own unsettled mind.

Two things could be causing a problem at this point in your yogic life. One is that the stimulating mental exercises may seem to have made it impossible to calm your mind, and secondly, you may have got such a new look at yourself that you begin to feel very alone and even more than a little frightened. It is to combat these thoughts that you can use Swami Hrydyananda's 'screen of love'.

The instructions given here are almost exactly those given by 'Mataji', as Swami Hrydyananda is affectionately called. Try if you can to have one room which is devoted to meditation and nothing else. It should be clean and devoid of distracting furniture. If you cannot manage to sit in one of the cross-legged Yoga poses comfortably–repeat *comfortably*–then you should use a chair. Make sure only that it is not too high and that you can sit with your spine as straight as possible. Sit with your hands loosely interlocked and your legs crossed because when you meditate you are generating a power something like electricity and you must prevent this current from flowing out through your extremities. Relax as much as you can while keeping the spine straight.

The first stage is one which you may have some difficulty with, but it is essential. Just close your eyes and allow thoughts to come and go in your mind at will. It is simply not possible to clear away all thoughts as soon as you sit down and begin to meditate. What you are doing at this stage is daydreaming rather than meditating. You should sit and build castles in the air, but it is not always pleasant castles that you will find yourself building. All sorts of thoughts will arise in your mind, pleasant and unpleasant.

Split your mind into two and let one part witness the thoughts which are passing through the other part. What have you done? The part of your mind which you have withdrawn is vibrating in a pure and subtle manner, while in the other part the thought waves are still crashing around. To calm the mind completely, you are going to allow the cool, soft vibrations to work on the rough, turbulent vibrations. As this begins to take effect, you may experience thoughts which are quite abhorrent to you. By watching your thoughts you have calmed your mind sufficiently to be able to see deeper into yourself and recognize some of the subconscious activity of your mind. These passionate unconscious thoughts have always been there, but until their release through Yoga you will never have been aware of them. All you need to do is watch, watch, watch, until they exhaust themselves. Keep a watch on them like an enemy but do not try to force them away and they will dissolve.

It is not possible to meditate properly until your mind has been cleared of these thoughts and this process may take some time, not merely one hour or one day but many days over many months. But even while learning you will benefit and become more peaceful. Above all do not worry about getting rid of thoughts. Simply relax and the relaxation will itself enable you to relax still further into your meditation.

At this stage it is worth going back to the physical and checking on the state of your body. Check that your neck, spine, and head are in as *comfortable* a straight line as you can manage, but under no circumstances attempt to sit to attention like a soldier. Gently close your eyes and let every muscle in the body relax, starting with the neck muscles. Mental tension causes most of us to sit with our shoulders slightly raised. So drop the shoulders. Work down your body literally from head to foot relaxing it consciously. Go through this routine two or three times until you are quite limp. Even your face must be relaxed. Do not hold your eyes shut too tightly or this will cause tension in the rest of your face and gradually spread.

Once again you are ready to sit and watch the thoughts go by. Now you should chant OM about half a dozen times (see page 68). For what purpose? Yogis believe that before the universe existed, there was only absolute consciousness. For anything to exist there had to be a vibration, and the sound of the word OM is the nearest we can get to this universal vibration. Chanting OM will bring you to a condition of internal peace in which you become open and receptive so you must ensure that the atmosphere around you is calm.

If you are facing the tensions inside yourself and beginning to relax them, you will become aware of the tensions or hate that exist in the world around you. To be able to complete your meditation you must have tranquillity. Like much of Yoga, the solution is so simple that at first some people tend to doubt it. You create an atmosphere of tranquillity simply by sending out thoughts of love, especially to those you think hate you. Hate only feeds on hate so thought vibrations of hate, worry, or tension which meet a screen of love can only dissolve or be turned back on themselves.

Of course you must be practical about this. It is no good plunging headfirst into a determination to gain peace through meditation and then rushing home and locking yourself in a room, having ignored your family and your friends. You must be sure that those near to you are made tranquil. There is no point, so to speak, in inviting attack.

So as you sit, first consciously send your love to those near you. Then gradually extend this screen from your family to include your neighbours, then the whole street, then the city, the country and the whole world. Let it grow until you feel at peace with the whole universe.

Now you are ready to get to the heart of meditation—to attempt a total stillness of the mind so that a superconscious state can arise. There are many methods but they all centre around the same idea, that you concentrate on some object until eventually your mind becomes so completely absorbed that it is "one pointed", i.e. it is conscious of nothing else but this one thing. To do this, you keep the object two or three feet in front of you and level with your eyes so that it falls into your field of vision when you are sitting comfortably. There are many objects which can be used, and among the commonest is the traditional candle flame. For the same purpose there are a series of visual patterns called 'yantras'; the word means no more than an aid. You can, if you wish, use a picture of your favourite teacher or a saint, but in this case you must gradually narrow down your vision until you

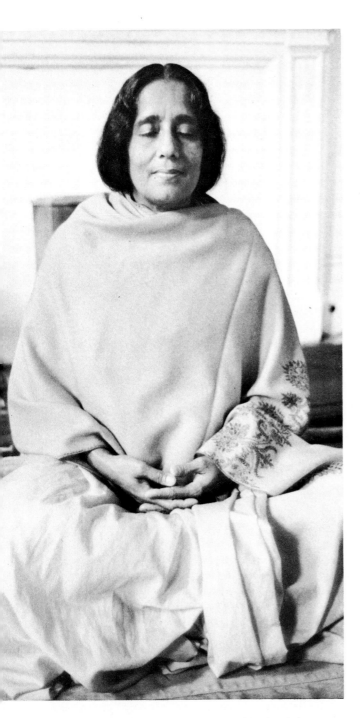

Swami Hrydyananda applies her 'screen of love' technique.

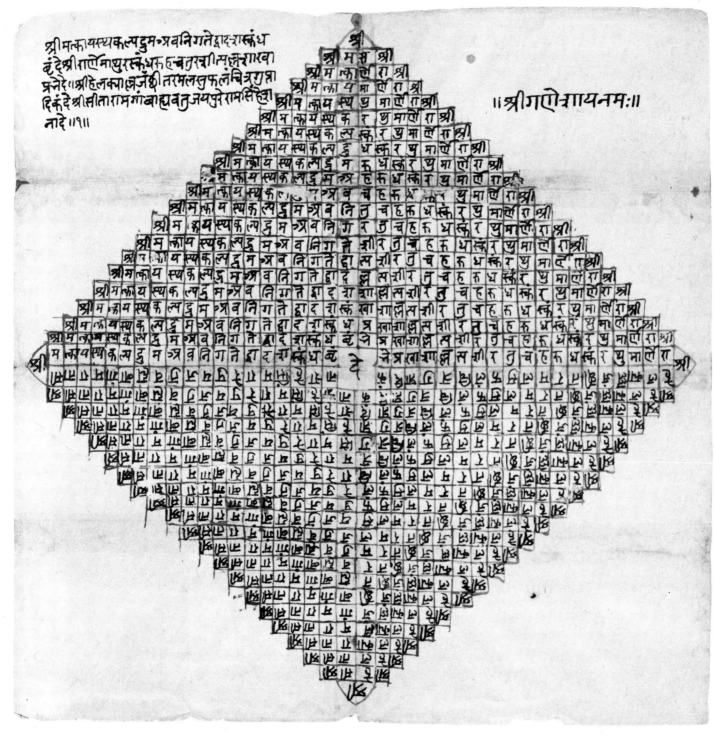

।।श्रीगऐैेरायनमः।।

Above: The Sanskrit alphabet has been formed into a yantra in this nineteenth-century drawing from Rajasthan.
Opposite: Eighteenth-century Nepalese manuscript with mandalas.

look only at one tiny portion of the picture, such as an eye or a foot. Whatever the object is, you stare at it without blinking for as long as you can without discomfort. When it becomes uncomfortable, you close your eyes and try to visualize what you have been looking at and you continue until you have the image firmly in your mind.

Once you have done this, then quietly, gently, and as slowly as possible, bring the image in towards you. It is important to avoid screwing yourself up with concentration. Keep your attention on the centre of the yantra or the heart of the candle flame but you *must* relax. You may still find that the occasional stray thought will pop up in your mind. Do not attempt to ignore it but just dissolve it as before, by watching it. Then return your attention to one pointedness. As you repeat this action, so such

thoughts become rarer and rarer. If you are successful with this technique you may begin to have a number of remarkable experiences. It is impossible to predict what any one person will experience but you may see strange colours and patterns, feel that you are floating in the air, or whatever. There is nothing to be frightened about in any of this. Simply continue to keep your attention on the one point.

Let us examine what is happening. In the beginning there were three things: first the meditator (yourself), next the process of meditation, and thirdly the object on which you were meditating. As your concentration becomes more and more

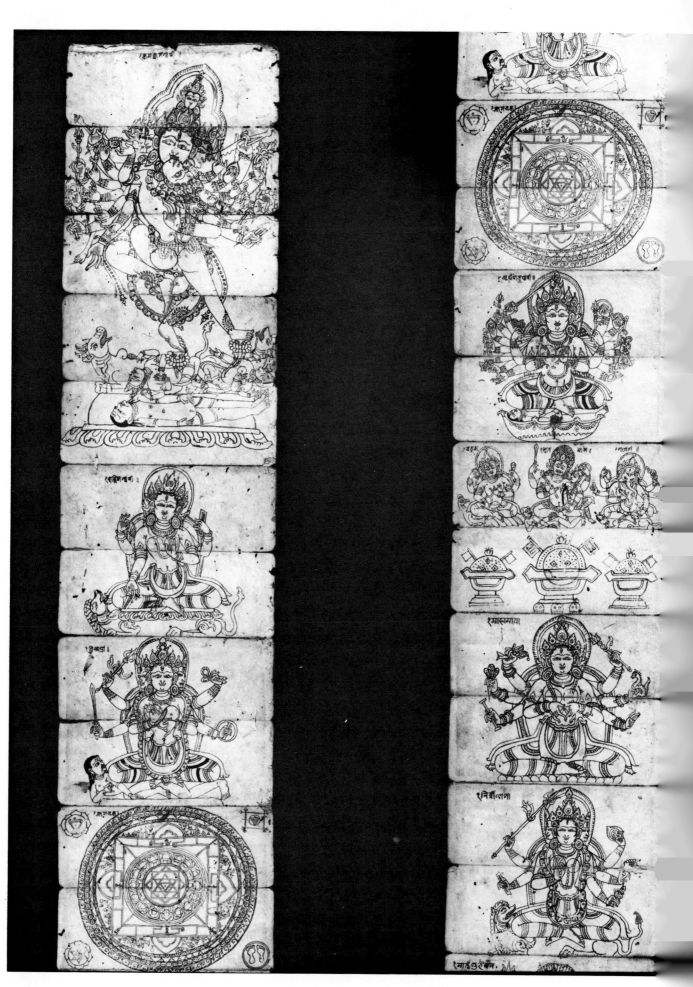

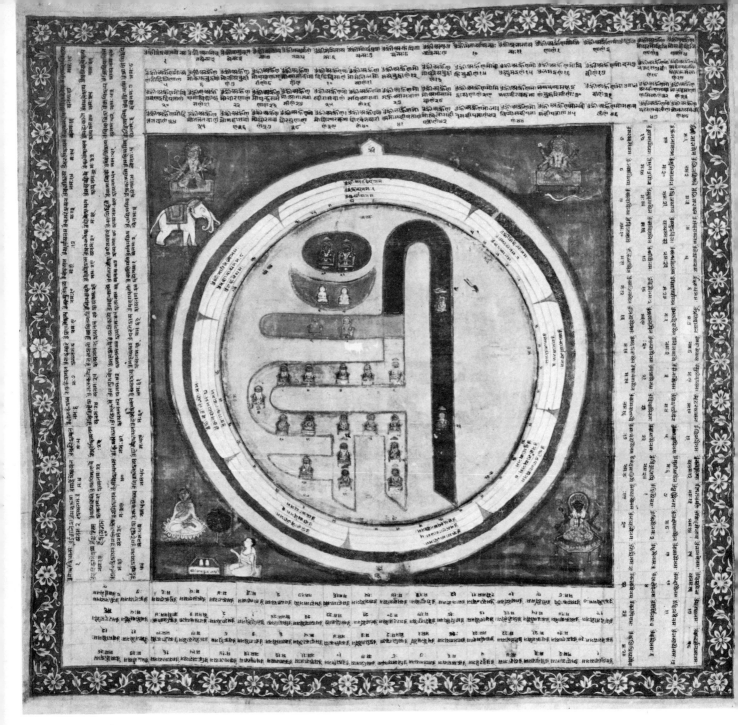

This Rajasthan yantra aims to create the sound OM in the mind.

powerful, the distinction between the three things vanishes. Every now and then you feel that you and the object you are meditating upon are one.

Then one day there will come a time when all the subtle energy units of the mind suddenly switch and you find yourself at one with the universe. This is 'samadhi', the superconscious state. Do not think, though, that after this you will have no use for the material world. Reaching samadhi is like tuning into a radio station; the choice of tuning into worldly consciousness is still open to you. And if you do tune back to worldly consciousness you have behind you the awareness of the other state so that you are no longer carried away by the conditions of the workaday world. You become more balanced, you lose your attachment to material objects, and you are able to live a peaceful life.

Some people are not able to cope too well with this process of inner visualization of objects, and

there is another technique for meditation which shifts the emphasis over to the use of 'mantras', or sounds. This is the technique advocated by the Maharishi Mahesh Yogi and it has been proved by laboratory research to be remarkably effective. The repetition of the word OM is in itself a mantra, but people are often given a personal mantra which enables them to achieve their one pointedness of thought and a cosmic vibration more easily.

A mantra may be chanted out loud but usually it is eventually taken inside the head, just as the visual image of the candle flame is, so that the chanting of the sound is a silent and inner sound. This appears a contradiction of terms but you can understand it very readily merely by humming a popular tune out loud and then humming the same tune silently inside your head. It is that simple.

'Yoga can only be known through Yoga'

Vyasa

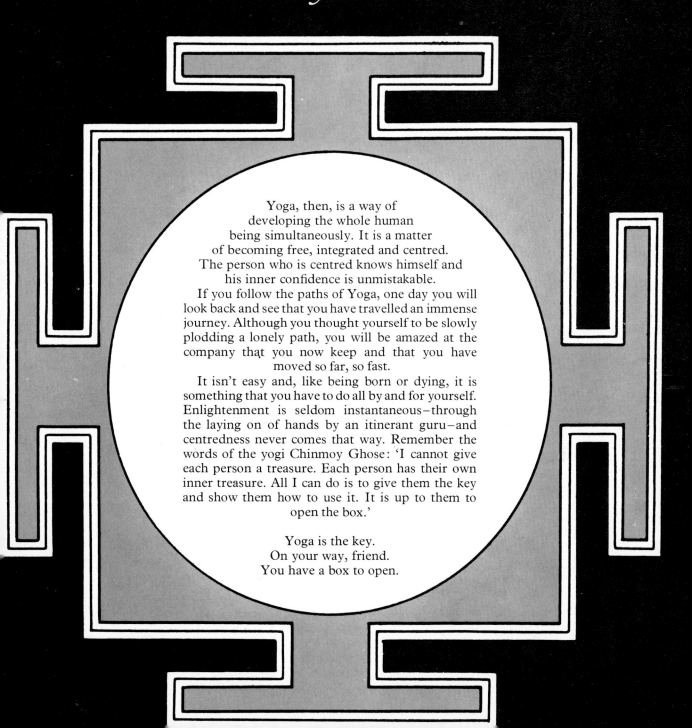

Yoga, then, is a way of
developing the whole human
being simultaneously. It is a matter
of becoming free, integrated and centred.
The person who is centred knows himself and
his inner confidence is unmistakable.

If you follow the paths of Yoga, one day you will
look back and see that you have travelled an immense
journey. Although you thought yourself to be slowly
plodding a lonely path, you will be amazed at the
company that you now keep and that you have
moved so far, so fast.

It isn't easy and, like being born or dying, it is
something that you have to do all by and for yourself.
Enlightenment is seldom instantaneous–through
the laying on of hands by an itinerant guru–and
centredness never comes that way. Remember the
words of the yogi Chinmoy Ghose: 'I cannot give
each person a treasure. Each person has their own
inner treasure. All I can do is to give them the key
and show them how to use it. It is up to them to
open the box.'

Yoga is the key.
On your way, friend.
You have a box to open.

bibliography

Priority titles

Fundamentals of Yoga by Dr Rammurti Mishra. Julian Press, New York, 1963. Lyrebird Press, London, 1972.
Light on Yoga by B.K.S. Iyengar. Schocken Books, New York, 1970. Allen & Unwin, London, 1971.

Suggested further reading

Be Here Now by Richard Alpert. The Lama Foundation, 1971, distributed in the US by Crown Publishing, New York, and in the UK by Neville Spearman, London.
Bhagavad Gita
The Complete Illustrated Book of Yoga by Swami Vishnudevananda. Julian Press, New York, 1960. Souvenir Press, London, 1961.
Knowledge of the Higher Worlds and Its Attainment by Rudolf Steiner. Anthroposophical Publishing, London, 1958, and Spring Valley, New York, 1961.
Occult Science: An Outline by Rudolf Steiner. Steiner Press, London, 1969. Anthroposophical Publishing, Spring Valley, New York, 1969.
The Primal Scream: A Revolutionary Cure for Neurosis by Arthur Janov. Putnam, New York, 1970. Garnstone Press, London, 1973.
Tibetan Book of the Dead edited by Dr W.Y. Evans-Wentz. Oxford University Press, London and New York, 1957.
Tibetan Yoga and Secret Doctrines edited by Dr W.Y. Evans-Wentz. Oxford University Press, London and New York, 1958.
A Treatise on White Magic by Alice A. Bailey. Lucis Publishing, New York, 1952, and London, 1963.
Yoga and Health by Selvarajan Yesudian and Elizabeth Haich. Harper & Row, New York, 1954. Allen & Unwin, London, 1966.
Yoga of Light: India's Classical Handbook by Hans-Ulrich Rieker. Herder & Herder, New York, 1972. Allen & Unwin, London, 1973.

INDEX

ACKNOWLEDGMENTS

The author would like to thank Georg Feuerstein for his help with the historical research, and Angela Farmer, Barbara Gordon, Nigel Hamilton, Lyn Marshall, Jacquie Perryman, and Peter Viesnick for modelling the postures.

The pictures listed here are reproduced by kind permission of the following collections and museums: British Museum, London 75; Chester Beatty Library, Dublin 87; Jean Claude Ciancimino, London 13, 121; Sven Gahlin, Sevington 11, 16; Gemäldegalerie, Dresden 27; Gulbenkian Museum of Oriental Art, Durham 99; Indian private collection 102–103; India Office Library, London 31; Musée Guimet, Paris 110; Museo del Prado, Madrid 94; National Museum, New Delhi 10; Tantra Museum, New Delhi 12, 35, 120, 122; Twentieth Century Electronics Ltd 36–7; Victoria and Albert Museum, London 18, 19, 28, 63 *right,* 95. The picture on page 49 is reproduced from L.A. Waddell's *The Buddhism of Tibet or Lamaism* by kind permission of W. Heffer & Son, Cambridge.

Photographic credits

Black and white

Archaeological Survey of India 10; Camera Press 7, 34, 93, 101, 108; Anne Cumbers 46, 47; Cuming Wright-Watson Associates Ltd 13, 121; Sally Curphey 21 *top left*; Mick Duff 43; Mark Edwards 6; Kenneth Grant 17 *top left*; Will Green 115; Gulbenkian Museum of Oriental Art, Durham 12, 16, 35, 120, 122; Hamlyn Group Picture Library, Derek Askam 42, 54 *bottom right*, 55 *left, centre* and *right*, 58–63 *left*, 64–5, 68–9, 70 *bottom*, 72–3, 76–7, 80–1, 84–5, 88–9, 105, John Howard 51, 106 *top left* and *right*; Graham Keen 41; Keystone Press Agency 56 *bottom*, 109; René Burri, Magnum 14–15, 100–101; Orbis, Derek Bayes 96, 97 *top* and *bottom*; Sally Patch 116, 117 *top, bottom left* and *right;* Picturepoint 45; Popperfoto 40, 57; The Ramakrishna Vedanta Centre 17 *top right;* Rex Features 39; Ben Rose Photography Inc., New York 20; Sri Aurobindo Society 17 *bottom right*, 24 *top;* United Kingdom Atomic Energy Authority 36–7; Victoria and Albert Museum, London 28, 63 *right*; Barbara Wace 24 *bottom,* 25; Edward Woodman 11; 'Yoga and Health' title page, 104, 119. The author supplied 21 *top right* and *bottom right,* 29, 32, 33, 53 *left* and *right,* 54 *top* and 56 *top left.*

Colour

Ampliaciones y Reproducciones Mas, Madrid 94; Mark Edwards 22; Gemäldegalerie, Dresden 27; Gulbenkian Museum of Oriental Art, Durham 99; Hamlyn Group Picture Library 19, Derek Askam 66, 67, 70 *top,* 71, 74, 78, 82 *left* and *right,* 83, 86, 90, 91, 111, Hawkley Studio Associates 75, John Howard 106 *bottom,* Rex Roberts Studio Ltd 87; Michael Holford Library 18, 110; Phoebus Picture Library 95, Robert Skelton 31, 102–103; Picturepoint 26; 'Yoga and Health' 23, 79, 98. The author supplied 30 and 107.